Mikayla's Journey

Kylie Henstock

Table of Contents

FOREWORD

My little girl,

All I want to do is protect you,

Keep you healthy and happy.

Sometimes I'm sure you're braver than we are.

One day I hope it all just stops,

But for now we just have to manage it the best we can.

Give you the best that we can,

We love you.

I am not a doctor. I am, in no way, an advocate for "doing your own thing." The specialists need to work WITH you to find the best way to treat what is happening. I was once told, "treating Epilepsy is more an art than a science," and I can vouch that this is true.

This story is my family's journey with Epilepsy, our daughters' journey. I hope it may help you and your family through your own journey. You are not alone.

All names of doctors, teachers and friends have been changed in this story to protect their identity. I've just kept my family's names true with their permission.

Chapter One

"Just move it slightly to the left," I said, "...a bit more...yeah that's perfect!" It was all falling into place.

My two young daughters and I were moving in with my boyfriend, Dave, and three of his four sons. Going from a small household and cooking for just me and the girls, to adding on four hungry males was a bit daunting. They were teenage boys with never-filling stomachs. But it was such an exciting move. Moving from small town Te Awamutu to sunny beachside Tauranga. I knew it would be a great change for the girls and me. We were moving from friends and family but it was only an hour and a half drive. Just over the hill, and we planned on making this work. I wanted to give the girls a stable childhood. No moving back and forth. We were determined to make our blended family work.

Dave and I had been dating for fifteen months. Long distance was hard but we saw each other every weekend with either him coming over to stay with the girls and I, or we came to him and stayed at his house with the boys. Dave has four sons aged twelve, fifteen, sixteen and seventeen. Aaron, the seventeen year old, had left home earlier in the year to study at University in Wellington. Dave and I had both been through divorces and were determined to give our relationship all we could. Neither of us had a lot of help with our children from our ex's. The girls loved Dave. He was fun and played with them even with their tea sets and Barbie dolls. It was so different for him from the rough and tumble of bringing up four boys, but he was loving the differences and taking it all in his stride. Mikayla was five years old and starting at the local primary school after Easter. Aleisha was almost four and would go to the close by day care centre for pre-schoolers. Dave's boys were amused with all the girly toys coming into their home. They had their own sleep out bedroom off the house so they had a bit of space from the onslaught. Ash was twelve and attended the local Intermediate school. Ryan was fifteen and Josh was sixteen, they both attended the College down the road. So our large blended family was nick-named the Brady Brunch by friends and it didn't take long before we found our feet and all got into a routine.

One night I cooked a cottage pie for tea. It was so big and heavy with all the mashed potato and cheese topping I could hardly lift it into the oven to grill the top. 'At least I'll have some left-over for lunch tomorrow', I thought. Little did I realise how much all these growing boys ate! The whole pie was eaten easily and I soon realised this amount of food was going to be normal for us to cook each night. It was crazy! So much food, so much washing and the toilet seat that was always up! All so different for me, but it soon became life and routine for us.

The girls enjoyed school and day care and loved having such a big family. There was always someone around to talk to and play with them.

It seemed to all be going well and we were all getting used to the household daily routine. I got a part-time job at the local MRI scanner. I was a Radiographer, but unfortunately couldn't find a job in Tauranga, so decided to take the training position in the MRI scanner. This was on the job training with two years of correspondence study through the University of Auckland. It was daunting with me being a not-very-computer-savvy, adult student, but Dave encouraged me, so I thought I'd go for it. Dave was a Real Estate Agent and could work around some of the school pick-ups when I was working, so it all fell into place.

Little did we know this three months of bliss was about to start us on the rollercoaster of our lives.....

Chapter Two

"Happy Birthday dear Aleisha, Happy Birthday to you!!!!...One, Two, Three, FOUR!!" we all sung. My parents had come over from Te Awamutu for the birthday party and Dave's parents who lived locally also joined us. It was a lovely evening and everyone got along well. Little Aleisha certainly enjoyed having all the attention and had a wide grin on her face the whole time.

"So how's it all going?" my Mum asked me. We were in the kitchen with Lyn, Dave's Mum, cleaning up the dishes.

"It's going well," I said. "I can't believe how much everyone eats and sleeps, but it's lovely to be able to see Dave every day."

"He's loving having you and the girls here too," said Lyn.

"You look so happy", Mum said, "I'm really happy for you, Kylie."

"Thanks Mum," I said as I hugged her.

"It is strange not having you round the corner though," Mum said. "Dad and I were thinking we could take the girls away for a night or two in the motorhome if that suited you?"

"Oh, they'd love that!" I said.

Everyone left later that evening with full stomachs and plans of the girls going with my parents in the next few weekends time for a break away in their motorhome.

Two days later I was shopping in town when I heard my phone ringing in my handbag. As I got it out I could see on the screen it was Aleisha's day care ringing me.

"Hello, Kylie speaking," I said.

"Kylie, hi its Annie here from Topkids Day care. I'm sorry to bother you but Aleisha has fallen from the monkey bars and appears to have hurt her leg. She's lying on the couch here now crying with one of our teachers. We've put ice on it but she's asking for you."

"Oh dear! Poor Leishy! I'll be right there!" I said.

I put the top I had been trying on back on the rack and went straight to my car. When I got to Aleisha she was pale, but not crying, and her leg looked okay, but she wouldn't weight bear.

"Thanks for ringing me," I said to Annie the teacher. "I'll let you know how we get on at the doctors."

I thought her leg would be fine but knew I had better get her checked over as she couldn't walk on it. It was two thirty by now so I thought I would get Mikayla from school on my way to the doctors. Mikayla's teacher was happy to let me take her early. At the medical centre we got through pretty quickly to see the doctor and he organised an x-ray just to be sure she had no fractures. I knew the Radiographer as she worked where the MRI scanner was that I worked on too.

"Kylie, do you want to take a look?" Sally asked.

"Sure, thanks" I said. "Oh crap!" I exclaimed when I saw the x-ray. A spiral fracture ran down my baby's tibia on the x-ray with a fracture through her fibula also.

"Gosh, she's been so brave! I honestly didn't even think it was broken! You'd think I'd know!" I cried.

"Happens all the time" Sally said. "My boy fell from the couch a few years ago, terrible broken arm and I had left him for a few hours with the ice-pack on it. He didn't even make a fuss. Honestly don't feel bad."

"Thanks Sal," I gave her a hug, "still, no more monkey bars for you for a while my little monkey," I said hugging Aleisha.

"What happens now Mummy?" asked Mikayla wide eyed.

"Well, Aleisha will need her leg to be put in a plaster by the doctor now," I said.

"Yes, come back round to the plaster room now," said Sally, "and I'll get the nurse and doctor to meet you there."

An hour later I walked out with Mikayla and Aleisha with a large white plaster on her leg going from half way up her thigh right down to her foot and a bright yellow wheelchair to wheel her in. I had bottles of Panadol and Ibuprofen to hopefully keep her pain at bay.

Dave was amazed to see how big the cast was even though I had rung him from the surgery, but it was still a shock. He carried Aleisha in from the car to the couch. She was heavier with the weight of the large plaster cast on her leg.

"Well, what have you been up to today? Thought you were a monkey I hear!" he joked with Aleisha.

"No Davey! I'm a girl, but I just slipped off the monkey bars!" Aleisha exclaimed.

"Oh I see," he said. "Well, you'll have to lay off the bananas for a while in case you think you're still a monkey!"

"Davey!!" she yelled. He was always joking and playing with the girls.

"Right, I'll get the washing in and start some tea," I said.

"No, it's okay I'll do it," Dave said. "You'd better ring your mum. She rung while you were out she'll be worried 'cause all I could say was you were at the doctors and Aleisha had fallen off the monkey bars."

"Okay. Thanks," I said.

I rung my mum and explained all that had happened.

"Oh gosh, poor Leishy!" Mum said, "Is she in pain?"

"Not at the moment," I said. "She's been very brave."

"Well keep up the pain relief cause if you don't the pain can build up quite quickly."

"Okay. Will do."

"Well, I was going to suggest Dad and I take the girls away in the motorhome on the eighth, but I guess now we'll have to see how Aleisha is." The eighth was a fortnight away.

"Yeah better just pencil it in," I said, "have to see how she goes."

"Okay. Well take care and I hope Aleisha is okay with no running round for a while," Mum said.

"True. I'll pop out tomorrow and get some activity books I think," I said. "She has some colouring in here, but good to get something new to keep her occupied. Bye Mum."

"Bye Kylie."

I went over to the couch and gave Aleisha a big hug. It's hard seeing your child hurt, but she seemed quite okay at present.

Over the next few days Aleisha managed quite well with the heavy plaster on her leg. She had some moments where it was very sore for her, but keeping the pain relief up for the first day or two helped her immensely. When it was time to transfer to a fibreglass plaster Aleisha chose a purple cast as it was her favourite colour.

She managed to move along the ground quite well on her bottom with her broken leg dragging behind her and whenever we went out she sat in her wheelchair while we pushed her around. Children are very adaptable to change and she took the days all in her stride.

In the end it was all fine for the girls to go away with my parents in their motorhome. It was decided a night away was enough. There was a bunkbed each for the girls at one end of the motorhome and Mum and Dad were in their double bed at the other end. Aleisha would sleep on the bottom bunk so it was easier to get her in and out with her broken leg.

The four of them headed off with lots of games and books on board and the wheelchair safely stowed away in the motorhomes underfloor garage. The girls left with huge grins as it was such an adventure for them to go away with their grandparents in the motorhome. Dave and I were also looking forward to a "date night" without the children around.

Chapter Three

The next day I got a phone call from my mum just before lunch.

"Hi," I said. "Is everything okay? How did last night go?"

"Not great," said Mum. "Dad and I have hardly slept."

"Oh no, was Aleisha sore or something?"

"No, it was Mikayla," said Mum. "She seemed to be having panic attacks all night."

"Panic attacks? What do you mean, what was she scared of?"

"Well, she would be asleep, "explained Mum, "then she'd wake up breathing heavily and trying to jump out of bed. She was on the top bunk and we were worried she'd hurt herself so we put her in our bed and Dad slept in the top bunk. She just kept doing it, over and over again. All night waking up and breathing heavily, trying to get out of bed, panicking about something. We put it down to anxiety from being away from you or something. But she did it all night."

I was completely confused and worried. She'd never done anything like this before. Here I was worried about Aleisha and her broken leg, and it was Mikayla who'd been the child with the problem.

"Okay, so when will you bring the girls back?" I asked.

"Probably about two if that's okay. I don't want Dad driving home late we are both exhausted from Mikayla's night," said Mum.

"That's fine. See you then," I said.

I hung up and went to explain the conversation to Dave.

"Sounds very strange," he said. "Maybe she was having bad dreams?"

"Yeah, maybe. But that many? All night?"

Mum and Dad drove up the drive just after two o'clock. They both looked exhausted and explained further about Mikayla's restless night.

"She seemed to be terrified each time," explained Mum, "and kind of making a sneezing type sound too, with wide eyes."

It really sounded strange but we had nothing else to go on so thought hopefully tonight would be better now she was at home in her own bed. Aleisha was fine and had enjoyed getting out of the house with a change of environment with her Grandparents. We said goodbye to my parents and waved them off.

That night we settled the girls into bed. They shared a large bedroom just off the lounge so we could hear them easily. They had both gone off to sleep and I could hear a noise coming from the bedroom. I went in and Mikayla on the far side of the room was in bed making a sneezing sound, then she sat up quickly and seemed to be panicking. Breathing heavily and trying to get the blankets off her and get up.

"It's okay honey," I said as I went to her. I held her and soothed her back to lying down. It lasted only a few seconds and she lay back down and fell asleep.

I went back out to the lounge to Dave and told him what had happened. We had only sat down for twenty or so minutes when she made the some sounds and when I went in to her the same things were happening. I reassured her again and lay her back down, soothing her as she calmed down and went back to sleep.

"It's like a panic attack or something," I explained to Dave. "Do you think she's worried about something at school, or being here, such a lot of changes for a little girl to process?" I was trying to work out what might be happening.

We got up to Mikayla ten times that night. But we ended up sleeping with one ear open for her so we felt exhausted when morning came and we hadn't had a relaxing sleep at all. Mikayla on the other hand was jumping round and happy like she normally was. A healthy little five year old.

That day after I had dropped Mikayla at school I rung Lyn, Dave's Mum to relay the goings on of the weekend to her. She explained perhaps its allergies. With us new to the area perhaps there's more pollens around. We also spoke about panic attacks and I said perhaps when she's asleep she's processing the move to Tauranga and it's upsetting her. New home, new school, new friends, new family……but we found this hard to believe as she seemed so happy with the new changes in her life.

That night about half an hour after going to bed, we heard Mikayla making the strange sounds she was making the night before. We both went in and Mikayla was sitting in bed, panicking and pushing the blankets off her legs. She was pale and breathing heavily. Aleisha was a heavy sleeper and just slept through the whole thing in the bed opposite Mikayla. We went to Mikayla and reassured her and calmed her down. After about twenty seconds she calmed down and we lay her back in bed where she fell immediately back to sleep.

We went back to the lounge and I picked up my laptop. I looked up allergies to pollens, cats and dust but none of the effects sounded like what Mikayla was doing. I also looked up panic attacks. Dave and I decided to take Mikayla to the doctor the next day to talk about things.

That night Mikayla had twelve of these "things" and again we were exhausted with the broken sleep.

We took Mikayla to the doctor the next day. They looked her all over and couldn't find anything wrong.

"It does sound like a panic attack of some sort," explained the doctor. "Keep to a regular bedtime, nothing too exciting before bed. Warm bath and quiet story. Hopefully it's just with all the changes she's had recently. She'll calm down soon."

So we followed the doctor's advice. Though we were already doing these things really. I had always ensured the girls had routine and were in bed early.

Once again that night, thirty minutes after I had put the girls to bed, Mikayla woke with panicked breathing, trying to get out of bed. We found her almost at the door when we got to her. Her little arms were flailing around, she was panicked with wide eyes and a pale face. I took her in my arms, but her arms were hitting my body with abandon, it was hard to hold her. Slowly she relaxed and her breathing resumed normality. I took her back to bed and lay her down.

"Darling, do you know what's wrong? "I said. I had tears in my eyes. I was afraid what was going on but I didn't want Mikayla to see my fear. Dave sat on the bed with Mikayla.

"Just relax Mikayla," he said. "Nothing can hurt you."

But Mikayla looked confused she had no idea what had just happened. I thought maybe it was a sleep walking type thing going on. We watched her fall back asleep and went back to the lounge.

"What do we do?" I said with anguish in my eyes. "She's obviously terrified about something."

"I don't know," said Dave. "Maybe we should take her to a Psychologist or something. See if she's worried about things that she feels she can't tell us?"

"Perhaps," I agreed.

That night Mikayla had fifteen episodes. I decided that was what I'd call them. I didn't like the word 'panic attacks.'

She had her school cross country the next day and the feeling of total exhaustion from the three nights we had had with little sleep were overwhelming. It was like having a new born again, but with worry attached to the tiredness. Mikayla on the other hand was oblivious to all this. She ran the cross country with all the energy of a healthy five year old. We stood on the side lines feeling drained and concerned but also thinking things can't be that bad. The doctor had found nothing and Mikayla looked absolutely fine in the daytime.

That night it was another restless night. Mikayla had five episodes before we had even gone to bed.

"I think we should start with the Psychologist," Dave said. "Then we can rule out anything that's mentally upsetting her. The doctors ruled out anything obviously physical being wrong."

"Okay," I agreed. "I'll ring around tomorrow."

The next day I made an appointment to see a Psychologist for Mikayla, myself and Dave. It wasn't cheap but we felt it was important to rule out any problems causing Mikayla's episodes which appeared to be so panic driven.

We got into the Psychologist two days later. We were absolutely drained and exhausted. We had had over a week with these disturbing nights now.

The Psychologist called us all into her office. She was a pleasant, softly spoken lady who had a lovely manner with Mikayla. She spent half the appointment speaking to us all and half the appointment just with Mikayla.

At the end she brought Dave and I back into the office and explained she would get a report of the session to us in the next few days, but that Mikayla was a normal, happy little girl. She could see no evidence that the move to Tauranga, new school or new family, was causing her any undue distress nor psychological turmoil. This was a wonderful result, but still left us none the wiser as to what was going on with her.

We thanked the Psychologist and left.

"What next?" I asked as we walked to the car.

"Not sure," said Dave. "Guess we just see how things go. Hopefully whatever it is goes away as quickly as its come."

That night Mikayla had fourteen episodes. They appeared to be getting more severe. She was even more panicked and flailing her arms even more vigorously. She made her way into the lounge for a few of the episodes. Her head looked up at the ceiling and she made choking sounds. It was terrifying to watch her. I held her little body and felt her heart pounding away in her chest. Slowly she regained her composure and I was able to sit her on the couch beside me. Once again she had no recollection of what had just happened.

The frequency of the episodes continued to stay high. Night after night she would wake with these panic attacks, always scared, always arms flailing, sometimes staring at the ceiling and this all lasted about twenty seconds, twelve to fifteen times a night.

Both our sets of parents were very concerned, but felt as we did, at least the doctor and psychologist found nothing so it can't be that serious. Our employers were noticing Dave and I were both very tired at work. The strange thing was Mikayla was not tired at all. Aleisha also was fine and was sleeping through everything every night. So were the boys as they were in their sleep out. Though they did see Mikayla having her episodes in the evening and were as scared and unsure as we were.

It was a very upsetting time and it was just the beginning.

Chapter Four

A week later we were still waking around fifteen times a night with Mikayla's episodes. During them she was running panicked through the lounge. More activity during each episode, more often than not her body would go rigid and she would tip her head back staring at the ceiling. Her heart pounding away under my hands.

"Enough!" I yelled after one particularly long episode. "I've had enough. I'm taking her to A and E."

It was two o'clock in the morning. The lack of sleep and worry for Mikayla had reached its maximum for me and I wanted a second opinion.

"I'm going to insist they let her sleep there so they can see what she's doing," I explained as I ran around finding Mikayla's dressing gown and slippers. "They just have to see what we've been seeing. It's the only way they're going to understand and work out what's going on."

I kissed Dave goodbye and bundled Mikayla into the car. I promised to ring Dave if I found out anything.

I parked in the hospital carpark and walked a tired, confused Mikayla into A and E.

"Hi," I said to the receptionist. "I need to see someone for my daughter please."

"Sure," said the receptionist. "What's her name? Date of birth?"

I gave her all the relevant details and we took a seat in the waiting room.

Mikayla's name was called about an hour later. She was tired and ready to lie down and have a sleep.

The doctor came into our room and I explained all that had been going on. He was very young and I felt like I was talking to one of my step-sons. But he was very nice and listened to Mikayla's chest, looked in her ears and throat and took her temperature.

"Well, why don't you rest in here Mikayla? I'll give you this alarm bell Mrs Henstock," he said. "Just press the bell if she has an episode and I'll be in as soon as I can. I'll let the other staff know what's going on too and if I'm tied up they can come in instead."

I thanked the doctor and settled Mikayla on the bed and dimmed the lights. I sat in the chair beside the bed and before long could feel my eyes getting heavy. Just then Mikayla sat bolt upright in bed her face terrified and pale. Her arms began flailing up and down at her sides. She was breathing heavily. I pushed the alarm bell the doctor had given me.

Mikayla stood up on the bed then and I had to hold her at the waist to stop her falling off the bed. She stood rigid and looked up at the ceiling making a choking sound. Finally a nurse appeared at the curtain.

"Oh my!" she said. "Help please!" she called to the other staff.

The young doctor who had seen us earlier appeared and watched as Mikayla continued staring at the ceiling with her rigid body standing upright and making the choking sounds. Slowly she regained composure and I was able to get her to sit down on the bed.

"So, is this the usual appearance of the episodes?" asked the Doctor as Mikayla came round.

"Yes. She usually gets out of bed panicking, flailing her arms around and runs through the lounge to us. Then she does what you just saw."

"Right, well from what I've seen it looks like a night terror to me," explained the doctor.

"A night terror?" I was surprised. "Okay, so what can we do about them?"

"Not a lot unfortunately. Children usually outgrow them as they mature."

"Oh okay, so we just have to get through this period….."

"Yes, sorry. I know that's not very helpful. Let me download some information for you and you can understand more about them."

So I got Mikayla off the bed and put her slippers back on her and waited for the doctor to return. He gave me several sheets of downloaded information and we left the hospital.

Dave was asleep when we arrived home again and I tried to slip into bed without waking him. He stirred and rolled over to see me. I explained what the doctor had said.

"Night terrors? Okay… so we just have to hope they go away as quickly as they came I guess."

"Yeah, I guess."

So we tried to get back to sleep, but part of me was waiting for the next night terror to have to deal with. My heart was heavy. It was horrible to watch Mikayla going through this. I could only thank the fact she was not getting tired from all this and it wasn't affecting her that we could see.

We continued on with family life and work the best we could. Aaron was back from University for holidays so it was lovely to see him again. Aleisha got her plaster off her leg and it was great to have her walking normally round the house again. Mikayla unfortunately was still having the night terrors every night. The frequency was still high with five to seven episodes occurring in the early evening and seven to nine from about three o'clock till morning. She seemed to sleep better from midnight to three o'clock and we didn't know why.

One evening Aaron and his friend Tony were sitting in the lounge with us watching television. The girls had gone to bed and suddenly we heard Mikayla panicking and running round in the bedroom. The door opened and she stood there pale faced and arms flailing. She ran around the lounge and saliva began running from her mouth. She stood rigid and stared at the ceiling saliva running down her chin.

Slowly she came to. Aaron had heard of what was happening but was shocked to see it in person. It wasn't nice to see this happening to your little step-sister.

"My Mum said I used to have night terrors," Tony said. Aaron had told Tony all about what we had been going through. "I outgrew them, though it was upsetting."

"Oh gosh, that's good to know," I said as I helped Mikayla to the couch and wiped her chin.

"Yeah Mum said I only had them occasionally. Once a night only and they lasted quite a while, like half an hour or so for me to calm down."

"Yes that's what I've read," I said looking at Dave. The information I had read on night terrors was that the child awakens from sleep panicked and even screaming. This terror lasts about one to two minutes but can last up to half an hour and the child usually has only one or two a night. This frequency and pattern hadn't sounded entirely like Mikayla's episodes to me when I had read the literature, but I figured maybe Mikayla's terrors were slightly different.

Over the next week Mikayla continued having her nightly night terrors, but they were becoming scarier. She would salivate each time now and occasionally she would wet herself. This did upset Mikayla as she had been toilet trained for quite some time and didn't understand when she came to why her underwear and pyjamas were wet.

I also noticed when her head was lifted up looking at the ceiling that occasionally her eyes would flicker. It was very subtle, but I said to Dave the first time I saw it, "It looks like a seizure, her eyes flicking like that," but I put it to the back of my mind as I had been told it was a night terror.

A night or two later I heard Mikayla starting to have a night terror. I went into her and was shocked by what I saw. She was still in bed, but instead of trying to get out she was on her back lying down. Her back was arched up and her arms were moving at her sides. She was making choking sounds and her eyes were flicking.

I screamed, it was a horrible sight and different to what I had seen her do before. As Dave came running to me Mikayla slowly came to. She began crying and I noticed she had wet herself. Her speech was slurred and I told her not to speak as I held her in my arms and soothed her.

"God, Dave that was a seizure I know it was!"

"What now?" he looked at me, "what do we do?"

"I'm taking her back to A and E. Things have changed. These are not night terrors."

We ran round getting clean clothes on Mikayla and a few bits and pieces. I put her in the car and kissed Dave goodbye.

"Ring me if you need anything hon," he hugged me tight. I could feel the tears coming again.

"I will, bye."

"Bye Mikayla, look after Mum for me okay?"

"I will Davey, don't worry." Mikayla's voice still had a slight slur to it. I was scared but feeling strong. I had to insist the doctors hear me and I knew in my heart these were no night terrors we were dealing with.

Chapter Five

We found ourselves in the same observation room that we were in a month ago. Mikayla was sitting up on the bed looking very confused.

"Is this because I wet myself?" she asked looking at me with big eyes.

"No my darling," I said giving her a big hug. "You can't help doing that. Mummy just wants the doctors to check out why you keep waking up in the night. Nothing to worry about."

"Do I have to have a 'jection?" she asked.

"An injection? I'm not sure sweetie. But if you do Mummy is here. I won't let anything happen to you." I was scared myself but definitely didn't want Mikayla to see this on my face.

The doctor came in then. She was slight and friendly looking and had a clipboard in her hand.

"Hi, Mrs Henstock. I've been reading what you told the Nurse. You have certainly been through the mill. I'm sorry about that. Hello Mikayla," she said directing her conversation to Mikayla. "How have you been little lady?"

"Okay," said Mikayla, "but I wet my pants and Mummy said it's not my fault."

"No Mikayla it's not your fault," she said with a smile. "I wonder if I could speak to you out here?" the doctor asked me.

"Sure," I said as I followed her outside the curtain. "Won't be long," I smiled to Mikayla. The Doctor took me into a room close by and asked me to take a seat.

"Mrs Henstock, it sounds like Mikayla may be having a type of seizure awakening her from her sleep. It may be that she's having two types of events. Night terrors and seizures but we'll know more after we run some tests. There are many types of seizures," the doctor explained. "Some occur while the person is awake, some while the person is asleep. If they occur only when they are asleep they are called nocturnal seizures."

"Okay. So what tests do we do to see if Mikayla has seizures? I guess you mean Epilepsy?"

"Yes Epilepsy," she confirmed. "Well, we need to organise an EEG that's a test where wires are placed on her skull within her hair and we look at the electrical activity in her brain. We can see if there's seizure activity occurring, we would also organise an MRI and perhaps look at putting her on an anti-epileptic medication if it was deemed necessary."

"Right, I actually do MRI scans so I understand that," I said. "You're looking for a physical reason she might be having the seizures?"

"Yes, it needs to be ruled out. I will speak to one of our Paediatricians in the morning and they will contact you with what happens next. You've done the right thing bringing her here," she said with a smile.

We went back to the room and she looked Mikayla over. As with other Doctors she could find nothing physically wrong with her.

We left for home again knowing we would hear from the paediatrician the next day who would organise the tests.

We arrived home and I updated Dave on everything I had learnt.

"Epilepsy….." he said.

"I know….. I don't think anyone in either of our families has it." It was certainly a lot to get our heads around. We both went back to bed for a few hours though we didn't sleep. We were trying to understand the diagnosis we had been told. It was hard to comprehend and it had come on so suddenly.

The next morning was a school day but I kept Mikayla home with me. She should've been exhausted with all the night terrors, seizures and time in A and E the night before, but she had lots of energy and kept wanting me to play games with her and read books. In the end I took her to the park and she spent the whole hour going up and down the slide. I could hardly keep my eyes opened by three o'clock when it was time to pick up Aleisha from Day care, but Mikayla was still full of energy. It was amazing.

At four o'clock my phone rung, it was a doctor from the hospital who introduced himself as Dr Downing, a Paediatrician.

"Mrs Henstock, I'm sorry to hear about Mikayla's recent turn of events. How has she been today?"

"She's been fine, full of energy. You'd never know how busy she'd been last night. It's quite hard to understand really." I explained.

"Yes, I'm sure. I would like to organise an EEG if that's okay. It would look at the electrical waves in Mikayla's brain and see if there's any seizure activity going on as some of the events you are describing don't sound convincingly like night terrors. Do you understand what an EEG involves?" he asked.

"Yes, the A and E doctor explained it last night to me," I said.

We spoke about meeting up after the EEG and going from there. He said I would hear from him when he had the results. He said we should get the appointment for the EEG within the next few days.

Four days later we were back at the hospital waiting for the EEG appointment. Mikayla was very brave and sat nice and still as the technician carefully parted her hair at regular intervals over her skull and wiped the area with a gel type liquid before placing a wire in place and securing it with tape. The wires took forever to get all in place and then her entire head was wrapped in a bandage to keep it all in place. Mikayla was encouraged to lie on a bed and the lights were dimmed. The technician took his place behind the console and tapped away for what felt like ages. He asked Mikayla occasionally to do a small activity. 'Close your eyes. Open your eyes. Cough. Blow on a windmill.' Then it was over and Mikayla sat up to get all the wires removed. Her hair was now a greasy mess, but the technician assured me the gel just washes out with shampoo. It would take time to look over all the data so we didn't leave with any results.

Two days later Dr Downing rung me. He said the results of the EEG didn't show anything conclusive.

"So she isn't having seizures?" I asked confused.

"She may be, it's still difficult to know. EEGs don't always show electrical changes with every type of seizure," he explained. "I would like to start her on a low dose of Epilim however, it's an anti-epileptic medication and may be able to stabilise things for you. We will need to do a blood test first to look at her Liver function before we begin the Epilim. I'll leave a form for you at the Paediatric clinic reception desk. I'll also send an MRI brain form through to Radiology though it may take a few weeks to get in for that."

"Okay, thankyou Dr Downing," I said.

Mikayla absolutely hated injections and screamed through the blood test. She had had thrombocytopenia - low platelets in her blood- just six months before we moved to Tauranga and unfortunately some of the blood tests for that were quite traumatic. Mikayla now had quite a fear of needles.

The MRI was organised a week later. I was able to speed things up by working with the Radiologists. Mikayla was amazing and lay perfectly still for most of the scan with me standing beside her holding her leg. The noises from the MRI scanner were loud and funny and I imitated them loudly to Mikayla trying to make it all seem less scary for her. She lost it by the end though. Half an hour is a long time to lie still for a young child.

Both the blood test and MRI results came back normal, but Mikayla was to start the Epilim anyway. She was still having the episodes every night with at least eight every night.

The Epilim came in a liquid form and was a red colour. I was told to measure it in a syringe and give it to Mikayla after breakfast and just before bed. It was a very low dose to begin with and I was told to increase it very slowly over the coming weeks until she was having five milligrams morning and night. Mikayla took the medicine well and never complained about the taste. I had a little on my finger one night and tasted it. It was horrible tasting and I thought she was doing great not noticing it.

Slowly over the next few weeks Mikayla's episodes slowly diminished. Firstly dropping to five a night, then two or three and then finally none at all. It was amazing!! The Epilim was a miracle medicine! We had our little girl back, not to mention our sleep. The change was so welcome. Dave and I had a new lease on life! It's so hard to concentrate when you're tired and I found work and study so much easier now. It felt like life was returning to normal.

Chapter Six

In August, four months after moving to Tauranga, Dave proposed to me. We had walked up the Mount to the most wonderful view in the area. He took me to one side and we looked out over the sea, the beach and down at the tiny houses and shops below. "I love you Kylie, and I would love to marry you if you would have me?"

"Of course I will!" I cried with tears in my eyes. Dave opened a small box and showed me a diamond ring. He removed the ring from the box and put it on my finger. I hugged and kissed him. I was so happy! We held hands and grinned all the way back down the Mount to our car.

Life was very happy and normal for about the next six months. We worked, played and slept! The children all enjoyed school and playing with their friends. Josh moved out. He had found a flat and started an apprenticeship as a mechanic. Mikayla started Soccer and Aleisha Ballet and they both enjoyed their chosen activities. There were no more episodes, and the Epilim seemed to be keeping things stable at quite a low dose.

We met up with a Paediatric Neurologist from Starship Children Hospital, Dr Hopping, who was doing a clinic in Tauranga. She was the guru in all things neurological with children. The Radiologists from work had told me how respected she was in the field. I certainly wasn't expecting this young, pleasant lady doctor. She was so lovely and easy to talk to. She was wonderful with Mikayla and had a great manner with her. Dr Hopping was pleased to hear how well the Epilim was working for Mikayla and examined her, finding nothing amiss. Mikayla had a mild eczema on her torso and legs and she prescribed some cream for this. She spoke about the episodes Mikayla had previously been having and said she felt these were never night terrors. She felt they were all nocturnal seizures probably frontal lobe due to the nature of them. Even though all the tests were negative she felt they were definitely seizures and wanted to order a repeat EEG this time sleep deprived. She said it wasn't urgent as Mikayla was now doing so well but would be good to get to complete the testing.

We left and felt very happy that things were good and on track.

The sleep deprived EEG was organised for a month later. It was very difficult to complete the preparation prior to the test, and Mikayla had to be kept awake two and a half hours over her bedtime and woken up an hour earlier than she would usually wake up. This meant she was easily asleep when she was on the table with the wires on her head and the testing was done with her asleep. Nothing happened as the Epilim was working so well now and we left with sticky, messy hair as we did last time. The results again showed nothing conclusive.

We looked forward to life resuming as normal. Mikayla's sixth Birthday came and went and we were looking forward to Christmas. Our first one in our home together as a big family. After Christmas we went on a camping holiday to Ohope and enjoyed a week in our tent. The boys in one tent, and Dave, me and the girls in another. We had a wonderful holiday.

January flew by and before we knew it Mikayla was back at school and Aleisha was back at Day care. Ash was starting at College with Ryan, and looked very smart heading off in his new uniform.

We had begun planning our Wedding for that September. We were planning an outdoor wedding by the water somewhere. As it was second time round for both of us it was more about friends, family and having a nice day than spending huge amounts of money on the day. Aleisha and Mikayla were very excited to be my flower girls and both started little wedding books cutting out anything to do with a wedding and sticking it in their wedding books.

Aleisha turned five in May and had a fairy party in our front lawn. Both sets of grandparents were there and Aleisha loved the Fairy Queen who turned up and took Aleisha and her fairy friends on an adventure of games and dancing. Our parents were so happy to see Mikayla so well and we just hoped the Epilim continued to work as well as it was.

In July, just when we thought the seizures were gone for good, they came back. Slowly at first, just a couple every other night, but within a month she was back to having clusters of three to five early on in the evening, and another three to five during the early morning. Her eczema seemed to get worse too and she seemed more anxious about school. I rung our paediatrician Dr Downing and explained the unfortunate change in events. He organised an appointment for us to catch up. He told us not to panic. Mikayla had grown and the small dose was probably just not enough now for her size. He told us how to increase her Epilim dose over the next month to get her on ten milligrams morning and night. Though if the seizures stopped at any point to stop at that dose so she was on the lowest dose possible to manage to seizures.

"Don't panic, it's just that she's grown since we put her on the Epilim. Increasing should contain things again," he said.

But increasing the Epilim dose didn't help. Mikayla continued to have nights of cluster seizures. Waking three to five times half an hour after going to bed. Running out to the lounge panicking, flailing arms and wide eyes, choking and dribbling. We would go to her and try and get her to relax but there was nothing we could do except wait the seizure out and ensure she didn't hurt herself. It was horrible to watch and there was nothing we could do.

Her school teacher was kept up to date with what was happening with her seizures and was very understanding. Then one day in August she asked to see me.

"Mikayla is slipping behind at school I'm sorry to say. It's not a huge difference from the other children but we're noticing her maths is most affected. Her retention is just not as good as it was," she explained.

This was obviously upsetting as Mikayla enjoyed school and had always been doing well till now. Though she was only young and I hoped we could get her seizures better controlled soon and her schooling would not be affected for long. Mikayla was also beginning to complain at the taste of the Epilim saying it was "yucky." Dr Downing organised Epilim tablets for Mikayla instead, and thank goodness she swapped to them easily, swallowing them with no problems.

Our Wedding was set for late in September. It was a beautiful, sunny spring day and we said our vows down by the water's edge in front of friends and family. Aleisha had been talking about 'walking in front of mummy dropping flowers as she walked' for almost a year, but when it came time to do her job she freaked out and ran off, and Aaron had to carry her up to the front with us. She took her place, as planned, but hadn't quite had the grand entrance she was looking forward to. Everything was perfect and the night had lots of dancing, beautiful speeches and tired children at the end. My parents had a room at a nearby motel and took the girls with them so Dave and I could have a night alone. The next morning everyone came to say goodbye to us and we went to the Coromandel for our honeymoon, leaving the girls to go to Te Awamutu with my parents for the week. It was the school holidays so no one was missing school. Dave's parents were there for the boys if they needed anything.

While we were away Mikayla continued to have her seizures and Mum and Dad were very tired when we returned to collect them.

"The seizures aren't being controlled very well we don't think," Mum said. "She's had up to ten every night we've had her."

"Yes, I think I'll contact Dr Downing, the Epilim isn't working as well as it was. Maybe we can increase the dose some more." We thanked my parents and went home.

I contacted Dr Downing the next day and he said I could increase Mikayla's Epilim dose a little more going on her recent weight. She could go to a maximum of twelve point five milligrams morning and night. He said that another medicine could be tried if that didn't work; Levetiracetam also known as Keppra. He explained he would contact Dr Hopping at Starship and update her on Mikayla. He wanted to see us in a fortnight to see how things were going. So over the fortnight we increased the Epilim to twelve point five milligrams morning and night, but it didn't make a lot of difference. Mikayla was still having eight to ten seizures a night and I explained that her schooling was suffering now also.

Dr Downing explained it may be time to introduce a second medication. If it helped then the Epilim dose could be decreased so Mikayla would be on as low a dose as possible to stop the seizures. Dr Downing explained to us how to start the Keppra tablets. Halving the tablets and starting with a half at night and building up to one tablet morning and night if required. These tablets were blue and bigger than the Epilim ones, but Mikayla swallowed them without complaint.

Then, just when we were worried about Mikayla and trying to sort out her medication, Aleisha gave us the fright of our lives.

Chapter Seven

It was early evening. I was studying at the computer in the dining room when I heard a funny sound coming from Aleisha's room, a banging, choking sound. I jumped up and ran to her room calling out to Dave. When I got to her door, Aleisha was lying in bed her left arm repeatedly bending and flexing at the elbow in a rhythmic pattern. Her hand was in a fist. Her head was also rhythmically jerking to the left in time to her arm moving. Her eyes were staring up at the ceiling glazed over and her face was contorted to the left. Dave drew up behind me at the door.

"No!" I screamed, "No!!" Not Aleisha too. What was happening to our girls? It was truly heart breaking. I sat on the bed with Aleisha trying to comfort her. It was obviously a seizure and it was just going on and on. She was trying to talk to us but the sound came out as a slurry incomprehensible sound. I was trying so hard to keep calm. I didn't want Aleisha to see me crying or upset.

Slowly over about three minutes, though it felt longer, her arm and head movements began to slow. Her face began to relax and she said "Muuuummmmy," very slowly and slurred.

I hugged my little girl and tried to reassure her that she was okay. Over the next few minutes her jerking had subsided and she sat up trying to talk to us. Her speech was very slow and her left arm just hung in bed beside her. She said it felt like a 'dead arm', not her arm at all.

"Oh darling! You're okay now, "I said hugging Aleisha hard. "We think you've had a seizure like Mikayla has." Though Dave and I looked at each other. Both of us knowing this was a different seizure than Mikayla has.

We took Aleisha to the lounge with us. Her gait was fine, but her arm was still hanging by her side. Her speech was getting better, but still had a slur to it. We sat down on the lounge suite with her and over the next few minutes her arm came back to normal.

"How are you feeling now Leishy," Dave asked her.

"I'm good Davey," she said.

"I guess we just ring Dr Downing in the morning and let him know what's happened," I said.

So we took Aleisha back to bed. She seemed back to normal now and happy.

She fell asleep again easily. Dave and I sat talking for ages. Comparing the seizures from each girls. There were similarities with them both occurring while the girls were asleep, but otherwise they were quite different. We went to bed hoping that Aleisha wasn't going to start on the same road that Mikayla was on, though knowing that this was a real possibility.

The next morning all was well. Aleisha had nothing untoward going on and could head off to school with Mikayla.

I rung Dr Downing's receptionist after I'd dropped the girls at school and told her what had happened to Aleisha the previous night. She said she'd inform Dr Downing when he was out of clinic later that morning. When he rung me early afternoon, he said it certainly sounded like a seizure, though probably not occurring in the same part of the brain as Mikayla's, and that was why the presentation of the seizure was different.

"How can both girls get this at the same age and there's no epilepsy in our families?"

"I would say it's a form of genetic epilepsy," Dr Downing explained. "I'll put in referrals for an EEG and MRI for Aleisha if that's okay."

"Yes that's fine," I said, "though Aleisha's a totally different kid when it comes to tests. I doubt she'll like the MRI, she'll probably need a general anaesthetic for it." From working in the area I knew some young children are terrified by the large machine and its loud noises, and require a general anaesthetic to remain still for the scan. I knew Aleisha would be in this category.

"That's fine, though as you know it will take longer to get your appointment is all."

"Yes, I know."

"So how has Mikayla been?"

"No change really yet. She's preferring the pills to the liquid," I said, "and we're still on the low Keppra dose. But she's still having seizures every second or third night. None last night."

"Okay, well increase the Keppra as I showed you, and please, ring if she gets worse or you have any questions."

I thanked Dr Downing and hung up.

Aleisha was fine for the next two weeks. There were no seizures and she was a happy little girl again. We were hoping it might've been a once off and were glad she didn't have the same frequency of seizures as Mikayla had. Her appointment arrived for the EEG, and they had gone straight for the sleep deprived EEG. Aleisha was such a different child though when it came to anything to do with doctors or hospitals. We didn't know why, but she was just so on edge and petrified, and it wasn't like she had had anything traumatic happen in her life. She was better at four when she broke her leg than she was now at five and a half. We followed the instructions of keeping her awake till ten o'clock, and that was difficult. She was such a busy child in the daytime and always crashed in bed at seven thirty so there was lots of book reading and games to try and keep her awake. Then having to wake her an hour earlier than she normally woke was also difficult. I felt cruel making her get up when she was tired.

When we got to the appointment Aleisha knew something was up. I hadn't explained too much because I knew she'd just panic, but I couldn't even get her to lie on the bed for the technologist. She looked at the screens in the room, trolleys and the stand with all the wires hanging off it and wasn't having a bar of it! She turned into one of those yelling, scared children who you just couldn't reason with. Everything I tried just wasn't working. There was no way Aleisha was having an EEG!

"They do give children a sedative sometimes," the tech said, "though it's usually for toddlers so I'm not sure."

"I'm so sorry, I thought I could get her to do this," I apologised.

The nurse spoke to us as we left, and told me we could try giving her some hydrochloride sedation first and trying again as it might be enough to relax her and get the test done. She explained it may not work though as Aleisha was a little bigger than most children they give it to. So Aleisha was booked in to go to the Children's Ward in two weeks to be given the hydrochloride sedation, and after it took affect they would try the EEG again.

I thanked everyone and left with my little monkey. She was exhausted from lack of sleep and all the tears and slept on the way home.

That night she was early to bed and we settled both girls off easily.

Mikayla woke with a seizure at eight thirty, running through the lounge with her usual panicked demeanour and flailing arms. She was dribbling and ran to the bathroom for a facecloth to wipe her face.

The cool, wetness of the cloth seemed to rouse her from the seizure faster too, though that may have been just coincidence. She was tired these days. Lots going on at school and this seemed to cause more seizures than usual also. The seizure stopped and we put her back in bed and she fell back to sleep quickly, as was usually the case. At nine o'clock she woke again and repeated the episode. The seizures always had the same appearance and lasted about thirty seconds. We had started keeping a record of her seizures, and times they occurred, so we could pass it on to Dr Downing when we next saw or spoke to him. I transferred the records into a 'seizure book' so we could compare nights and see any trends.

Then at nine thirty, we heard Aleisha having a seizure. It looked just like her last one. She was lying in bed with her left arm jerking rapidly, bending at the elbow with a clenched fist. Her head was jerking again too. The seizure lasted about three minutes and she came to with a slurring to her speech and a lifeless left arm. Again she came right over the next five or so minutes. It was certainly scaring us how our nights were changing into caring for our newly epileptic daughters. It was upsetting, and we felt on edge for when, or if, a seizure would occur.

Mikayla slept a few hours after that and then had four seizures in quick succession from three o'clock. We found that these cluster seizures stopped if we 'broke the cycle' of them. We would take her to the lounge and read or watch television with her. This seemed to work and she wouldn't have any more seizures for a while if at all.

I rung Dr Downing the next morning and told him of our busy night. He was sorry to hear that Aleisha had had another seizure and said we should go to the EEG appointment as arranged. He arranged to meet up with us in clinic following the EEG. He said as Aleisha's seizures were different to Mikayla's and lasted longer, we needed to be mindful that if they lasted five minutes or longer we were to ring for an ambulance. This was scary to hear but I understood. He also said the MRI under general anaesthetic had been organised for a months' time, just to rule out any physical reason for the seizures. We spoke of Mikayla and he arranged to meet us with both girls in a week so we could talk about things.

The day of the hydrochloride sedated EEG arrived and we once again followed the instructions of the sleep deprived EEG. I was certainly very familiar with the routine by now! We arrived at the children's ward at the specified time and we were given an area of the preadmission clinic with a bed. A nurse arrived and took some obs on Aleisha and gave her some books and games to play with. Aleisha was scared, but so tired she didn't mind the nurse taking her blood pressure and pulse recordings. Hopefully this time things would work out I was thinking.

An hour later the hydrochloride sedation was given to Aleisha in a drink form which she didn't mind taking. Nothing seemed to happen for the first ten minutes, then Aleisha needed the toilet. She was so dizzy and wobbly on her feet I had to help her walk to the toilet and go. On walking back she was even more unsteady, if that was possible, and I picked her up to carry her back to the bed. But she suddenly lashed out and flung her arms around and arched herself backwards. I could barely hold onto her. I got back to her bed and lay her on it and she yelled and thrashed around I could hardly hold her on the bed. A nurse came in and said the sedation did this sometimes and aggression was common. Together we tried to stop Aleisha falling off the bed and hurting herself. We didn't want to put up the side bars as she was lashing out and she would've hurt herself. She was only five years old but she was strong at that moment! As suddenly as it began, it stopped. She lay down with her head on the pillow and calmed right down. Within a few minutes she closed her eyes and began snoring. It was weird stuff this sedative! The orderly arrived a few minutes later and took us down to the EEG department. The tech from last time said "hi" and proceeded to get ready to start placing the wires on Aleisha's head for the test. He was about a quarter of the way though and had to move Aleisha to get better access to her head when she stirred and opened her eyes. I spoke softly to her encouraging her to close her eyes again, but she wasn't having a bar of that and sat up suddenly her head pulling on the wires that had been placed in position. She screamed as they pulled on her hair and that was that.

"Oh dear, Aleisha, come on sweetie relax and let the man finish. It's not going to hurt you…" I tried to encourage her to continue but she was not having it.

Unfortunately, second time round was also a no go. I couldn't believe we had spent all morning trying to get this test done but had failed again. There was no reasoning with Aleisha she'd made up her mind and was not happy about this.

I apologised profusely to the tech, he had wasted another appointment on us but he assured me that it wasn't rare and some children just couldn't comply. I didn't know what this meant for helping treat Aleisha's seizures but I couldn't do anything more today, so home we went.

A week later we meet Dr Downing at his clinic. We had both girls with us and I had the seizure book with a record of seizures in it. Dr Downing said although Aleisha had not had the EEG the week before not to panic, it wasn't vital and we'd just continue with the MRI as planned and go from there. He examined her and found nothing untoward and spoke of starting Aleisha on the liquid Epilim that Mikayla had been on to begin with. He said as she had had two seizures now, he felt a low dose would be necessary to start with. He arranged a blood test to ensure her liver function was normal prior to beginning the Epilim. I knew that would be fun to get with Aleisha but said I'd buy some numbing gel. With Mikayla he said to continue increasing her Keppra dose as we still had a way to go. He noticed that her eczema was a little worse and gave us a prescription for some steroid cream, he also noticed that she hadn't put on any weight for a while and asked about her appetite. I said I hadn't noticed anything different and we spoke about her decline at school also.

We thanked him and left.

We continued on as usual, Mikayla still having seizures two to three nights in a row with cluster seizures on these nights. We didn't notice any trends really, but did see she had more seizures if she was anxious about something coming up like the school cross country, or excited about something like Christmas or a birthday party. We noticed both girls had seizures if they were tired too so kept their bedtime routines very strict to try and alleviate this. Aleisha was having a seizure about once every five weeks and they were always in the early evening while she was asleep. She tolerated her Epilim well and didn't fuss at all over it so that was good.

The day she had her MRI went fine. I knew everyone there and knew the routine. Aleisha turned up at the appointed time with a hungry tummy having had nothing to eat all morning. She sat on my knee in the prep room as the anaesthetist placed the mask to her mouth. She suddenly realised something was happening and began to yell and thrash about on my lap, but the gas took effect quickly and she became limp in my arms. The medical staff lifted her from me on put her on the table and I left them to look after her to complete the anaesthetic and MRI scan. It was very different being on the other side though, and I would lie if I said I wasn't anxious. Finally they came and got me to go to recovery as Aleisha was waking up. She awoke upset and a lemonade ice block was brought for her as soon as she was able to have it which soon quietened her. The results of the MRI were normal which was a great relief and again pointed towards looking like a genetic form of epilepsy.

Chapter Eight

The end of the year approached and I had completed my studies in MRI. It was a great relief to be over and we ensured we all could get to my graduation ceremony.

Time passed and Aleisha's seizures seemed to be well controlled on the Epilim. She was up to seven point five milligrams morning and night and hadn't had a seizure in some time. Poor Mikayla on the other hand, had been on the maximum doses of both the Epilim and the Keppra for her weight, and the seizure control wasn't great. In fact the seizures were now increasing. She was eight and a half years old and her seizures were occurring nightly, with some nights having as many as twelve seizures. We would spend parts of the early morning watching up to fifteen minute blocks of children's television to try and break the clusters of seizures.

Lyn and Colin, Dave's parents, would have the girls for a night or two over the odd weekend just to give us a reprieve from the broken sleep. It was certainly starting to take its toll on our health, both physically and mentally. During the school holidays Mum and Dad had the girls in Te Awamutu for a few days. Mum rung panicked one morning saying Mikayla had just had a seizure at the breakfast table.

"Was she asleep at the table?" I asked confused.

"No, she was awake. Eating. She said 'I feel weird' then started breathing strange and panicking. Like she does with a seizure at night. She got off the chair and continued having the seizure like she normally does…”

“Oh no, not in the day too now….”

I hung up and couldn't stop the tears. This changed everything. To me we could cope with the nocturnal seizures, but daytime seizures seemed to put another twist on things to me. Made it something others would see and judge her on at school and if we were out. It was just horrible for me to get my head around.

I contacted Dr Downing's receptionist. I felt it was important for him to know this new change in events. He wasn't too concerned when he contacted me back later that day. “It can happen with seizures unfortunately,” he said.

So we just carried on, Mikayla not getting any better and Aleisha doing fairly well on the low dose Epilim.

The next time we had our appointment with Dr Downing he was not happy with her weight and said her growth had stagnated. He organised an x-ray of her wrist to look at her bone age which came back normal. He said the seizures at night are interrupting her sleep which is when she's growing, so it can affect her growth. Also the medications can affect her growth so he wanted to keep an eye on this. Her schooling was starting to suffer more too and she was slipping further behind.

Dr Downing contacted Dr Hopping from the Starship Children's Hospital to see what else could be done, and she suggested looking into trying a new medication, Tegretol, also known as Carbamazepine, if things didn't improve. Two months later with Mikayla now almost nine years old, there were further concerns for her seizure control. They were increasing in frequency each night, and beginning to last longer each time, up to a minute long each. Her weight and height were also a concern with still no increase in quite some time.

Mikayla started on a low dose of Tegretol and saw a decrease in seizures within days. After four days on the Tegretol her seizures stopped and we were so excited and thought we had found the medication to finally stop all this, but it was short lived. Ten days later the seizures came back and she was having five to seven per night again. This rapidly increased and one night we just couldn't get the seizures to stop. She would close her eyes and ten to fifteen minutes later would be up having a seizure. She would try again to sleep, and again, a seizure. It was cruel and relentless. Finally at ten thirty I said to Dave, "she's had twelve already, I think we need help." I took her into A and E. I explained what was happening, and they soon saw her have a seizure when she fell asleep beside me on a chair in the waiting room. The other people in the waiting room looked pretty shocked, but anything goes in that place really. After what felt like an eternity talking to one doctor, retelling it all to another, we finally made it to the Children's Ward. The paediatrician on call came into our room and I relayed it all to her. Dr Singh was just lovely and could see the worry in my face.

"You've certainly been through it by the sounds. Unfortunately Mikayla's seizures are tricky to control. Obviously, there are drugs we give some children to stop them seizing, but Mikayla's seizures aren't Grand Mal seizures or unstoppable as far as each seizure goes. But the frequency is the problem. Settle in this room for now and I'll contact Starship and see what they say. It may be we don't get an answer till morning though." I understood.

A nurse arrived and took Mikayla's obs and gave me a seizure chart which I was to fill out with each seizure she had. I was to record the time, how long the seizure lasted, what she did, and her appearance throughout. I settled us in for the night and it was busy. Eighteen seizures by morning and that didn't count the twelve she'd had at home. I was exhausted by morning and Mikayla looked worse for wear too. The Paediatrician came in at nine o'clock and looked at the seizure chart.

"I haven't heard from Starship yet but I'm sure they'll get back to me this morning," said Dr Singh.

"Thank you," I said.

That afternoon Mikayla looked exhausted. She was pale and withdrawn.

"Let's try and have a rest baby. You and me," I said. I took her into our room and pulled the curtains. She drifted off to sleep within five minutes and awoke ten minutes later having a seizure. She ran into the main corridor of the children's ward and was choking and panicked. Her arms flailing by her sides. Her legs stomping on the hard linoleum floor. People watched her and tried not to stare, but it was a busy time in the ward and Mikayla was very loud. I tried to take her back into our room and slowly the seizure stopped and I took her back to bed. But my tears came. I was tired, scared and thinking 'will this stop?' I turned away from Mikayla I didn't want her to see me upset. But I couldn't contain myself. I left the room and just bawled. The receptionist looked up and came over to me.

"It's okay," she said. "Nicky, can you look out for Mikayla?" she asked a nurse. "Mum and I need a walk," and I let it all out. The worry I had for my little girl and whether this was all going to stop and the exhaustion Dave and I were feeling. She was amazing. She took me to a room for parents of patients and made me a hot drink. She just listened and when I finished she said, "I can only imagine what this is all like for you all, but they're not going to send you away until you've got some reprieve so take all the help you can here…" She led me back to my room and my little girl.

Dr Singh came in to see me an hour later. Starship Hospital had contacted her and wanted us to try intravenous Midazolam. "I'd like to connect her to a monitor when the Midazolam is given just to check everything is okay. Hopefully it will slow the seizures down and give her some sleep," she told me.

The Midazolam was connected to her intravenous line with a machine which dripped it into her body slowly. Mikayla was so exhausted she slept as it went in and she managed to sleep an hour and a half with no seizures. It was wonderful. Unfortunately, the

Midazolam only worked well the one time, and when it was given again later that night it had minimal effect on stopping the seizures. Mikayla had another busy night with seizures.

"Are you sure you don't want me to come up to the hospital?" Dave asked me the next morning when I told him about our night.

"No, you get Aleisha and the boys sorted and come up later," I told him. Dr Singh was at the door of our room. "I have to go honey, Dr Singh is here. I'll talk to you later, bye." I hung up.

"Hi Kylie, "she said. "I heard last night wasn't good. I'm sorry to hear that. I've heard from Starship, we're going to start you on a new drug called Clobazam. It's given at night only with her night medications, so we'll start on a low dose tonight and go from there."

"Okay, thank you," I said.

The Clobazam was given that night with the Epilim, Tegretol and Keppra and worked straight away. Mikayla had a wonderful night's sleep, and we were discharged the next day.

We went home and it was so lovely to see everyone and have the home comforts again.

Chapter Nine

Two days later Mikayla had her end of year dancing rehearsal for hip hop which she had been learning. As I watched Mikayla dancing on the stage, she looked so small and pale. I sat beside Louise, one of the other dancers mums' and told her of Mikayla's recent admission into hospital. She couldn't believe how many seizures Mikayla had been having when I told her.

"Well, hopefully this drug is the one. All the best," she said as we left after the girls rehearsal. That night Mikayla slept well again.

The next night was show night and Mikayla looked so tired and pale but she was insistent that she wanted to do the show. I was so proud of our girl. She must've been exhausted but she just carried on and wanted to do her dance. Dave, me, Ash, Aleisha and Dave's parents were all there to cheer her on. We were very proud of her.

Ten days after we had started on the Clobazam, the seizures started again. We couldn't believe the Clobazam wasn't working either. I ran into my friend, Liz in the chemist while I was filling out a prescription for Mikayla.

"Kylie, how are you?" she asked hugging me.

"I'm fine," I lied. Liz had known me most of my life, we had been friends back in Te Awamutu from the age of five. She looked into my face and knew I wasn't telling the truth.

"Oh Liz, it's just horrible. Mikayla is just not responding to the medications. Well, she is at first and then it's like her body works out how to fight back and the seizures start again." Then the tears flowed, I just had so much pent up worry for Mikayla and seeing Liz just brought it all out.

"Come on, let's go get a cuppa and you can tell me everything," Liz said. It was lovely to talk to her and she was shocked how bad things had gotten. I think a lot of our friends didn't realise just how bad it was for us, and we didn't want to complain to everyone.

Four days later we were back to seizures every five to ten minutes. They just didn't stop. We tried breaking the seizures by getting her out of bed to watch television, or to read, but we also were just so tired it was hard to stay awake with her. We decided to take her back into Hospital.

I packed a bag, grabbed her medications, and kissed a fast asleep Aleisha on the cheek. That was the hardest thing for Aleisha to understand. She goes to sleep and wakes up and her Mum and sister have gone to hospital for days at a time.

I kissed Dave goodbye and gave him a fierce hug.

"It will all be fine soon…" he said. Though the look he gave me was one of worry and extreme tiredness. We had hope that this time things would work, but it seemed the seizures were testing the doctors' skills too. We arrived at the hospital and went through the usual hours in the waiting room and A and E until we got to the Children's Ward. The paediatrician who saw us was an older, South African man, Dr Forbes. He had a gentleness about him and kind blue eyes. Even though he had Mikayla's previous files in his hands he wanted me to retell her last few years. He listened intently and said, "I definitely think Mikayla needs to be seen at Starship if possible. The number of seizures she is having is getting concerning. Let me make a few calls and I'll come back to you. Settle in here, this is your room for the rest of tonight." He stood and left the room, pulling the door behind him.

The nurse came in a few minutes later with the seizure chart I recognised from last time for me to fill in. She took Mikayla's obs and I settled her down into bed for what was left of the night. The seizures started again within ten minutes and the nurse came in to help and watch Mikayla. She had another seizure ten minutes after the first.

"Oh my gosh! It's just so frequent!" she said touching my arm. "How have you all been managing this at home? Honestly it must be so hard on all of you."

"It has been. But what else do you do?" I said. "It's just been getting through the best we can."

"Well, I think you've done amazing," she said. "Truly, it must be so tiring. Dr Forbes is really good though. He'll get things organised. Honestly, he's really passionate about cases like yours."

I thanked her and settled Mikayla down again for what it was worth. I knew she'd be seizing again soon. It really was so worrying.

Dr Forbes came in about an hour later and I told him she'd had six seizures since we'd last seen him. He shook his head.

"Well, I've got through to Dr Sharon Pope from Starship she's on call tonight. Do you know her?" I shook my head. "I've told her all about Mikayla, and she said if you can make it to Starship Hospital in Auckland tomorrow morning by nine o'clock they will do a Video EEG on Mikayla tomorrow night. Just by coincidence they have a service on the machine tomorrow morning. It's an automatic software download which starts at three o'clock in the morning, and they hadn't booked anyone in the room because of it. Because Mikayla's seizures are so frequent I think they'll get a lot of information about her seizures during the day tomorrow and up to the three o'clock cut off time for the download. They will also then be able to help with medications to get the seizures better controlled. You'll be with the best doctors to get this sorted. Now can you get in Auckland by nine o'clock tomorrow morning?" It was eleven o'clock and I agreed, saying I would ring my husband straight away. I thanked Dr Forbes and picked up my mobile.

Dave answered after a few rings, he was asleep.

"Of course, I'll take you both," he said. "I'll ring Mum and see if she can come and get Aleisha tomorrow morning. The boys are here till she gets here. Poor Leishy, she's going to be upset. She didn't even get to say goodbye to us all."

"No. I know. But we have to go. The waiting list to get this video EEG is months long apparently. We're so lucky to get in so fast."

"Yeah, no it's meant to be. Right. I'll ring Mum now and pack a bag for Aleisha. Do I stay in Auckland with you?"

"Yes, please. I'm exhausted. I think we need to be together. Take turns with Mikayla. Hayden and Teresa would let us stay with them if we asked I know they wouldn't mind." My brother and sister in law lived in Auckland.

"Okay, do you or Mikayla need anything else from home?" he asked.

"No. We'll be okay. I'll just buy anything we've forgotten. What time will you be here in the morning? The traffic will be horrible getting into Auckland." It was a three hour drive from Tauranga to Auckland and with the traffic we didn't want to be stuck in a traffic jam and arriving late.

"Four thirty…five….earlier the better. I'll go now. Ring Mum, pack and try and get some sleep. Good luck for tonight babe. Just get through tonight and they'll help us up there…."

"I hope so Dave. I love you. Thanks for sorting everything there."

We hung up and I went to find Dr Forbes, letting the nurses know I wasn't in with Mikayla in case she had a seizure while I was out.

"I'll pop in with her," our nurse said.

"All set?" Dr Forbes asked when I saw him.

"Yes. My husband, Dave, will pick us up early tomorrow morning."

"Perfect. Here's the directions to get to the Neurology Ward. They're expecting you at nine o'clock and will take you down to get Mikayla wired up for the EEG. Okay?"

"Yes. Thank you so much for organising all this Dr Forbes," I said. My eyes began swimming with tears. I quickly blinked so they didn't fall but I wasn't quick enough and I swiped them away with my hand.

"You will get some answers up there Mrs Henstock. It's the best place to be. They will help you."

"Yes." I nodded. "Thanks again," and I went back to Mikayla and our room.

"No seizures. She's asleep." The nurse said when I returned. "Are you all sorted?"

"Yes we're going to Starship first thing tomorrow morning," I whispered so as not to disturb Mikayla sleeping.

"Good. They're amazing up there!" she said. "I've worked there about five years ago when I got home from my O.E. The staff are so caring and it really is the best place to be when you're in a situation like you're in. They will help you."

"Yes, everyone is telling me that. Thanks so much."

"Try and get some sleep. Ring the bell if you need anything. I'm due off my shift soon, but all the best and I hope you're home again soon with things much better."

I thanked her and tried to settle down for sleep. It was a horrible busy night with Mikayla though and before I knew it, it was time to get up and shower to be ready for Dave to pick us up. I found our new Nurse for this shift and told her I was having a quick shower and could she listen out for Mikayla.

At four thirty Dave arrived, and Mikayla and I were dressed and ready to go. Dave didn't look much brighter than us and we said we'd stop at the nearest service station for coffees. We thanked the medical staff and left with the papers we had to hand over to Starship when we arrived.

Chapter Ten

The drive to Auckland went well though Mikayla had two seizures in the car when she fell asleep. One just before we hit the motorway and one on the motorway. I hated it when she had seizures in the car. Dave slowed down and pulled over if he was able to. We always locked her door because we were afraid she might go for the door handle during a seizure. I just reassured her the best I could and waited till the seizure stopped.

We drove in to the Starship / Auckland Hospital just before eight thirty. It had been a long drive, but we did well to get through the morning motorway traffic and had just had a quick stop to get coffee. We followed the instructions to the Starship carpark and found an empty park. We unloaded and followed the instructions to the Neurology Ward. The hospital looked so amazing, nothing like a hospital. The atrium of the hospital had a merry-go-round, which a young boy was on even this early in the morning. The tinkling cherry music echoed in the atrium. We looked up and saw a high round wall of pastel coloured floors. Each colour indicating a different floor in the children's hospital. Two glass elevators moved up and down the circular floors. You could see the people within each elevator as they moved up and down to get out at their designated floor. It truly was a magical first sight of this place, which we hoped held all the answers to help our daughter.

"Wow!" said Mikayla looking up. "Is this a hospital?"

"Yes. It's pretty cool aye," said Dave.

"Yip." Mikayla took my hand and we walked through the atrium to the glass elevators. We took the elevator to the floor with the Neurology ward and went through to the reception. We told the lady there who we were and she said, "Won't be long." She spoke into a microphone and her voice echoed through the ward.

"Helen to reception please. Helen to reception."

As we waited for Helen, we looked up and down the corridor from where we stood. The ward was in a horseshoe shape with the reception in the bend. The nurses and doctors congregated behind reception in a large room and the patients rooms came off the corridor off each side. Breakfast was being served to the children in the rooms by a lady pushing a large metal trolley.

A tall, thin lady walked up to us and introduced herself as Helen.

"Hi, you must be Mikayla, I'm Helen," she said smiling at Mikayla. "Hi, I'm the Charge Nurse in the Neurology ward," she said to Dave and I. "How was your drive up?"

"It was fine," I said. "Thank you so much for fitting us in today. We really appreciate it."

"It's worked out well. Come this way. This is the room we do the video EEG's from." She took us just a little down the corridor into a room on the left. I noticed the room number was thirteen. The room had a bed and a screen hanging from the ceiling from the front of the bed. Behind the bed were lots of wires going down the length of the wall. A bathroom was visible just off the room. There was a table and a sink also in the room.

"So, this is Mikayla's room for today and tonight. We'll take her down shortly to get wired up for the EEG, then she'll stay in here till tomorrow morning. We'll be able to monitor her here the whole time, looking at her electrical brain waves, and also watching her on the camera while any seizures occur. Your job Mum and Dad, will be to squeeze this alarm bell with each seizure which will alert the Neurologist that a seizure is beginning when they look through the tape. Also making a note of the seizure on this chart," she said showing us a chart very similar to what we had been using in Tauranga Hospital. "So, make yourselves at home. The bathroom is here." She said indicating the bathroom off the room we were in. "Mum or Dads bed is here," she indicated what I thought was a wardrobe, but it was a bed hidden away upright into a closet type cupboard. It took up hardly any room and had a big thick mattress looking very comfortable. "Come this way. I'll show you where the linen is kept for your bed and towels. There's a kitchen this way for you to make hot drinks and there's bread where you can make toast for breakfast." The kitchen window had a wonderful view right down into the atrium of the hospital. I could see the merry-go-round way down below. "There's a play room this way for Mikayla, but she'll be wired to her room for today so she'll only get here from tomorrow," she said walking further down the corridor and showing us the room off the other side of the corridor where a few children were playing inside. "So relax for now. An orderly will come and get you from your room just before ten to take you down to get Mikayla wired up. Are you okay with that Mikayla? You've had an EEG before in Tauranga. Do you remember what that's like?"

"Yes, I think so," Mikayla said.

"Great. Well, I'll leave you now. Is there anything else you want to know for now?"

"No, I don't think so," Dave said.

"Good. So I'll see you when you get back from getting wired up," she smiled and left us.

We got a cup of tea each and wandered back to our room. Mikayla asked if she could play in the playroom and we said yes we'd come and get her when it was time to go down to get the wires on. We were just discussing ringing Hayden and Teresa and seeing if one of us could stay tonight when a nurse came in.

"Hi, I'm Katie. How's it all going?" she was a very smiley girl with olive skin and her hair pulled back into a pony tail.

"Its fine thank you," I replied.

"Great, now where's wee Mikayla?"

"She's playing in the play room. Shall I get her?"

"No, she's fine for now. I just need to do her obs and put her patient identification on her wrist. Now, when are you going down to Ronald McDonald house to book in there?" she asked.

"Um, I didn't know we were going down there," I said. "I was just about to ring my brother and see if one of us could stay there."

"Oh no. Ronald McDonald house is on the hospital grounds and so much easier for you. Did you get booked in there from Tauranga?"

"Um, not that we know of," I said looking at Dave.

"This was all organised very quickly," Dave said.

"Right. I'll ring and see if I can get a room for you. Shall we go and see Mikayla and then I'll ring for you?"

"Okay," I said and followed her down to the play room.

She came back to our room about half an hour later and said, unfortunately, Ronald McDonald House was full. Both houses had no rooms available for the next two nights.

"That's okay I'll ring my brother," I said.

"No, I've spoken to the Charge Nurse and we have a few spare rooms down the far end of the ward. You are welcome to take turns when you're not with Mikayla to sleep down there. It'll be much easier to do the swap overs and you won't need to drive when you're tired. I also have these vouchers. Show them to the car building guy when you leave and it's a set rate of five dollars per day otherwise it'll cost you a fortune."

"Oh that's so lovely of you. Thank you," I said. I couldn't believe how helpful and lovely everyone was here.

Just before ten o'clock an orderly came and collected Mikayla. I went with her and Dave was taken with a volunteer for a walk round the hospital. They showed him where the Ronald McDonald Family Room was. It was a place we could go for time out, and where food was donated to families by local businesses. Salad rolls and fruit were there, and Dave was allowed to take some for our lunch. It was a truly humbling experience and when Dave told me about it when we met up later he had tears in his eyes. The kindness of others when you're tired and worried about your family is a really emotional experience.

Mikayla was very good at the EEG department. The technician measured her skull and carefully applied each wire to her scalp with the special gel and tape just as she'd had done in Tauranga. It was a very slow, precise job and when it was done her head was wrapped in a gauze bandage to keep the wires safe from movement. Then all the ends of the wires were placed in a velcro sock which had a special connector at the end where all the wires were inserted.

"Then this is plugged into the machine back in your room," the technician explained to us.

"She gets up and runs during her seizures," I explained to him confused. "How will the wires reach without pulling out?"

"The plug in the room has a pretty long cord," he said. "She'll be able to run round her room without dislodging anything."

"Okay, thank you very much," I said.

The technician led us back to our room at Starship which I was grateful for. The department we were in was in the depths of the Auckland Hospital and it was confusing to get back to Starship Hospital. I knew I would've gotten lost.

He asked Mikayla to climb into bed and he took the connection which held all the ends of the wires and plugged it into the matching connector from behind the bed. This had a long cord attached so Mikayla, in effect, had a long cord coming off her head which followed her if she needed to use the bathroom or had a seizure. We would just need to make sure she didn't trip or get caught up in anything with it.

I thanked the technician and he left.

"Well, that's you now for a while honey," I said to Mikayla. The play therapist had brought in a CD player with lots of CDs, books and games for Mikayla so she could entertain herself from the room. Mikayla was now on a CCTV type get up, with her image appearing on the screen ahead of her so the doctors could visualise her seizures when she had them. The rest of the day was spent just hanging out in the room. I rung my parents and updated them on our sudden change of plans. They were obviously shocked that we were suddenly in Starship, but really happy that hopefully things would get sorted for Mikayla. Dave made a few work calls and rung the boys to check things were good there. Ryan said that Lyn had arrived at nine o'clock to get Aleisha and that Aleisha was confused and worried. I rung Lyn's and updated her and thanked her so much for getting Aleisha at such short notice.

"I don't know how long we're here for Lyn. How are things there?"

"Everything's fine. Don't worry. Do you want to talk to Aleisha?"

"Yes please. Thanks Lyn."

"Not a problem. Here she is….Aleisha, mums on the phone for you," she called.

"Mummy? Hi," Aleisha said, "You'd gone when I woke up."

"Yes. I'm sorry sweetie, there was no time to talk to you. Everything happened when you were asleep. Mikayla is in a special hospital just for children up in Auckland now. We'll be back as soon as we can. The doctors just need to try and stop Mikayla's seizures so we can all have a good sleep at home. Okay?"

"Yes, okay. But I miss you….." I could hear her voice cracking.

"I know. And we all miss you too honey, but Mikayla needs the doctors help and then we'll be home as soon as she's better okay? I'll ring you every day and tell Nana to ring me if you need me okay." It was hard to explain things to her, but I hoped she understood. "Now you go and be a good girl for Nana and

Grandpa, and we'll all be home as soon as we can okay?"

"Yes, I'll be good. Bye Mummy."

"Bye sweetheart." I hung up and blinked hard. The tears were stinging my eyes. It was so hard to be away from her, especially as we hadn't had time to say goodbye, or explain things to her properly.

At seven o'clock Mikayla's eyes were getting heavy, so we got her to brush her teeth and got her into her pyjamas. Her tops had to all have button through fronts so they could come off, as the wires didn't allow anything to go over her head.

"Right. All ready for bed Daddy," said Mikayla sitting up in bed with the unusual headgear dominating her small body in the bed.

"Right. Well say night to Mummy, she's going to go down the corridor and have a sleep,"

"Okay. Night Mummy."

"Night darling." I leant down to give her a hug and kiss goodnight. "Mummy will come in later. I'll just go and have a sleep for a bit first," I explained. "Thanks honey," I gave Dave a kiss.

"Now you take as much sleep as you need. Don't hurry back. We're fine here, aren't we Mikayla?"

"Yes," Mikayla nodded.

"Okay, well see you later." I went to the room we had been given for a much needed rest. It had been a long day and I was exhausted. I fell asleep within minutes and awoke with my alarm just after two o'clock. I was disorientated and it took me a moment to remember where I was, and why. I got up and straightened up the bed, though Dave would be back in the bed soon. I put on my shoes and walked through the quiet darkened corridor towards Mikayla's room. I looked through the glass in the door and saw Dave sitting on the parent bed by Mikayla's. He looked shattered and smiled at me.

"Hi," he whispered as I opened the door.

"Hi. How's it been?"

"Pretty bad. She's had well over twenty seizures already. The nurses were coming in every time I pushed the button for the video but I've told them we're fine and they don't need to. They can't believe how many she's having and how often.'

"Yeah, I bet," I said. I took a look at Dave's chart. He had already filled in the first side of the paper and was on to the second side.

"Well, you go get some sleep babe," I said. "I honestly feel so much better now."

"Okay, night hon." He gave me a kiss and left to go down to the room.

He hadn't gone long when Mikayla had a seizure. I pushed the button and jumped up to help her. She bobbed up and down on the bed with her arms flailing beside her. Her face was contorted and panicked looking and she was making loud choking sounds. She started getting off the bed and running towards the bathroom. I had to make sure she didn't trip on the long cord coming off her head. The seizure lasted about a minute, then she slowly calmed down again and I took her back to bed and settled her down. I wrote on the chart, the time, how long the seizure was and what she did and just put my pen down when she started again. I pressed the button and did it all again. The nurse appeared in the doorway and shut the door behind her. She smiled with a concerned look on her face and helped me manage Mikayla. When the seizure finished she helped me get Mikayla back into bed.

"Hi Kylie. I'm Tracey. Sorry I didn't get in to see you earlier it's been a busy night."

"It's fine. I just swapped over with Dave. He did the night up till just a while ago."

"Yes, I met him. Such a busy time you both have had at home with Mikayla like this. How have you managed?"

"It's been hard. Hard to get up in the morning when you're exhausted. Poor Mikayla. Each morning we have to decide if she can go to school and sometimes it's hard to get her out of bed. She's getting very little sleep. Hopefully the doctors have some answers for us here," I said.

"Childhood epilepsy is such a tricky thing to manage," Tracey said. "But yes, hopefully they can help you…."

Tracey stayed and talked for a bit longer then she left me with Mikayla. The rest of the night continued to be busy, and by six thirty Mikayla had had forty-four seizures. I couldn't handle her having anymore. The video EEG had stopped working by three o'clock anyway for the planned service, and they had thirty or more seizures captured on the video. I made her stay awake and turned on the lights. I turned on the CD player we had been given from the play therapist and selected a CD for her to watch. I decided to go and make myself a cup of coffee and ran into Tracey in the corridor.

"How are you?" she asked.

"I'm fine. Just going to make myself a coffee. I've woken Mikayla now she's had enough seizures. At home we break up the clusters up if we can, but it's tricky when we're in hospital. I guess it's good to get lots of seizures on the video for the doctors to see."

"Yes, she's certainly given them a lot to look at," Tracey agreed.

I said bye and continued to make a coffee.

It's weird being awake early in a hospital. Walking the quiet, darkened corridor when everyone is asleep. The odd room has a crying child or a nurse taking obs by flashlight, but otherwise it's an eerie time of the day. You're tired and your senses are on high alert. Extreme tiredness makes your sense of touch and sound far more sensitive, and you almost flinch at high pitch sounds, or if something touches you.

I made my way back to Mikayla with my coffee. Slowly the ward woke up and we could hear children and parents moving round in the corridors. Staff were walking around and the day shift started. Dave came in looking dishevelled and tired at eight o'clock.

"Hi. How'd she go?" he asked.

"She had heaps. They've got lots to see," I told him. "When she got to forty-four I kept her awake."

"God, that's so many," he whispered running his hand through his hair.

It really was getting scary and I was so thankful we were in Starship.

The doctors did their rounds about nine o'clock and it was so reassuring to see our Neurologist we had met in Tauranga, Dr Hopping, leading the team around the ward.

"Hi," she acknowledged us. "Hi Mikayla. Do you remember me? I met you and Mum and Dad at Tauranga Hospital a while ago. Do you remember?"

"Yes," Mikayla smiled and nodded. It always amazed me how alert Mikayla was after such a terrible night of seizures and lack of sleep. Although she was pale, she was alert and happy.

"Right, well it definitely looks like we've got lots of seizures to look at on the video. It will take a few days for me to go through and watch it all. Now, looking at the medications she's on at present, I think we should stop the Keppra while you're here. It's not really helped at all. I would like to start her on a new medication. It is called Phenytoin. It's actually one of the older drugs, but if we do a loading dose tonight we can see if it's going to help at all. I would also like to organise an MRI scan. I know she's had one before but that was on 1.5T and as we're looking for such a tiny focus our 3T scanner may pick that up, okay?"

"Yes," we nodded.

"We can do things quicker with the medications while you're here. Loading and stopping the medications while we can monitor Mikayla and see how she is."

"Great, thank you. Dr Hopping, have you seen seizures like this before? This....frequent?"

"Yes I have. It's not a common type of seizure to have, and the amount Mikayla is having is rare, but hopefully we'll find the drug to settle things for her. So far the respite from seizures has been short-lived with the Clobazam and Tegretol, so hopefully we find something that keeps them away for longer."

We thanked Dr Hopping and her team, and they left to continue their rounds.

"Phenytoin," I said writing it down. I liked to look on the internet what the drug was like and the side effects it had. All the medications had its own list of unpleasant side effects. It was just a matter of finding one which worked to alleviate the seizures, while not having too detrimental side effects. This one had dizziness, drowsiness, confusion, nausea, vomiting, tremors, slurred speech, and loss of coordination, amongst other things.

We had breakfast and got Mikayla dressed. A lady came and removed all the wires from Mikayla's head and carefully wiped the gel from her hair. Her hair was sticky and sticking up at all angles, so I gave her a shower and washed her hair. We were moved to another room as the video EEG room was needed for another child to be monitored today and tonight.

Dave went and made some work calls, and rung the boys to make sure all was okay at home with them. I rung my parents and Dave's parents and had a chat to Aleisha. I also rung work and updated them with what had happened, and they gave me the rest of the week off to be with Mikayla, saying if I needed more or got back earlier just to ring and let them know. They were very sympathetic and understanding of our situation, and I was very grateful. Mikayla's school were also so supportive and sent best wishes to Mikayla. We spent the morning filling in time in the playroom. In the afternoon, my brother Hayden, his wife Teresa, and their three children Zach, Dylan and Hannah visited us. It was lovely to see them, and the children kept themselves entertained playing. They loved watching the air ambulance helicopter taking off from the helipad and landing which we could see from our bedroom window.

"How are you going?" Teresa asked me, she was sitting on the end of the bed with a cup of tea.

"We're worried and tired obviously. But this place is the best place to be. They'll get her sorted," I said.

"Yeah, and the nurses seem so lovely," Teresa said.

"They are. Nothing is too much worry. They even organised a bed down in a room for us last night, and they've offered it again tonight. We'll have a room in Ronald McDonald house they said, the night after that."

"That's wonderful. You know you're more than welcome to stay at ours too."

"I know. Thank you."

"How long are you in for have they said?"

"No. They want an MRI while we're here….and to get the medications sorted so the seizures are more manageable."

"Well, anything you need, anything at all, just yell out," she said.

"Thank you," I said hugging her.

The men just walked in with the entourage of little children.

"Hi Mummy, we went on the merry go round!!" yelled Hannah to her mum.

"Wow! Aren't you lucky!" said Teresa.

"Ky anything you need, I was saying to Dave, just yell out," said Hayden.

"Yes, we will, thanks so much," I said.

We had a lovely afternoon together and they all left late afternoon.

That night we got Mikayla settled for bed and the doctors came in with her medications. The loading dose of Phenytoin was a lot of capsules for her to swallow, but she managed well. She also had her Tegretol and Epilim, but they had stopped the Keppra.

We were given a seizure chart to fill out as before, but didn't need to worry about any recording tonight.

"Still, use the alarm bell if you need anything, or if you're worried," our nurse said. "I will check in on you too."

We thanked her and I gave Mikayla a hug and a kiss and went off to my room down the corridor for a sleep. Although it was only seven thirty I fell asleep straight away and awoke at one thirty with my alarm to go and swap with Dave.

"Do you need more rest? I'm feeling okay," Dave said when I opened the door.

"No, I'm feeling much better. I flaked out straight away," I said. "How's she been?"

"Not great," Dave replied. "She's had twenty-two already."

"Well, that Phenytoin doesn't look like it's done much then," I said sadly.

"No, and she's pretty wobbly too when she gets out of bed. You have to keep an eye on her or she's liable to fall over."

"Okay. That's no good."

I hugged him and he left to go down to the room for a sleep.

The rest of the night was busy, another eighteen seizures, and by quarter past six I decided it was time to keep her awake. Out came the CD player, and the lights were turned on. You have no idea how hard it is to read a book when you're tired. Television and CD players are a godsend and I don't care if it sounds bad. It was easy and entertained her to stop falling back asleep. She was just so wobbly I had to hold her up and carry her to the toilet. She couldn't walk at all. Her speech was slurred and difficult to understand. I was very concerned and so were the nurses. They saw our light on when they walked past and came in.

"How's our Mikayla this morning," Hayley the nurse asked, giving me a knowing look.

"Gowd," she slurred.

"Sometimes the Phenytoin can do this," she explained to me. "Obviously the doctors will look her over when they do their rounds, but just keep an eye on her if she's getting up, and ring the bell if you need a hand with anything."

"Thanks, I will," I said.

She left and I sat on the parent's bed watching Mikayla, who was watching the television. She looked pale and exhausted. About half an hour later she said "I seal stick," and looked even paler, if that was possible. I jumped up and just got to her in time with the vomit container. She wretched uncontrollably and emptied out her stomach, poor little thing. She threw up till she had nothing left, and no energy to vomit anyway. I lay her back on the pillows and put the container on the bench. I wiped her mouth and forehead with a cool wet facecloth and rung the bell. "She's just thrown up," I told the nurse when she arrived in the room.

"Oh poor poppet," she said coming over to Mikayla. "Are you feeling better now Mikayla?"

She smiled at the nurse but she looked terrible. "I might just take her obs if that's okay," she said.

Everything was fine with the obs. "I think it's the Phenytoin," she said. "I'll page the doctor and let them know she's not well, but I think we just have to wait for the medication to get out of her system. I could get them to organise something for the vomiting too."

"Okay, thanks." I said.

Dave came in at seven o'clock and I retold him what he'd missed. "Oh poor thing," he said.

She needed the toilet again and couldn't even stand. Dave lifted her in his arms and carried her to the toilet. It was horrible to watch her unable to walk, talk and feeling so rotten. He carried her back to bed when she'd finished and went to get us both a hot drink. Later he was brushing his teeth and I was texting, when in the corner of my eye I saw Mikayla falling. I reached for her, but was too late. She fell out of bed, her little body hitting the floor hard. She didn't put out her arms at all to stop the fall and her head hit the ground. I screamed and ran to her. As I lifted her I saw blood streaming from her mouth and she was crying loudly, disorientated. Dave ran to us from the sink and lifted Mikayla to her bed again. The nurses came running to our room they could hear Mikayla and me crying. I was beside myself. I just wasn't myself at all. Seeing my child in this way unable to help herself and now with blood pouring from her mouth, I was hysterical. Hayley tended to Mikayla with Dave, and I had to leave. I sobbed blindly down the corridor and found a room just a few doors down. I'm normally a rational, sensible woman, I would say, but at that moment I was broken. I needed to get away. I couldn't care for and protect my daughter. She was going through hell and I couldn't help her. I was so tired and so worried. As I sat in one of the chairs my head was in my hands and I just couldn't stop crying. I felt someone sit beside me and an arm went round my shoulders.

"It's so hard seeing our children going through this, I know," said a kindly, older woman's voice. "If we could change places with them we would do it in a heartbeat aye?" I nodded and tried to calm down and wipe my eyes. "It's okay to be upset, and it's okay to let it out. I would say it's important, or you won't get through it, okay?"

I looked at her she was a round, kindly faced, elderly Maori lady. Her arm was so comforting around my shoulders, and she handed me some tissues.

"Thank you," I said taking some from her. "She just fell from the bed, there was blood ….and she doesn't need this…she's going through so much already," I hiccoughed.

"We all have a breaking point," she said. "This was yours. Take some time and when you feel better you can be strong for your girl again, okay?"

"Yes…okay. And thank you so much. I'm embarrassed to have lost it like that…."

"No….as I said we can only take so much pain…..you're her Mum and you need time for you too." She took her arm away and stood up smiling as she walked out. She was like an angel to me that day. I hope she knew what a help she was.

Dave came in then. "You okay?" he smiled.

"Yeah, sorry. How is she?"

"She's cut her lip. The doctors are looking at her now. They don't think it needs stitches, and her teeth look okay at the moment. Still all there and not broken."

"Thank God," I said standing up. Dave came and gave me a hug. "Come on she needs us," and he lead me out of the room.

When we got back she was sitting up in bed with a swab on her lip held with tape and big tears still in her eyes. I went to her sitting down on the bed and took her in my arms. "Darling you okay?" She nodded and tried to talk. "Just rest for now Mikayla. We'll keep the sides up on your bed today just in case okay," and again she nodded. We had a quiet day. The doctors came to see us on their rounds and looked Mikayla over. Dr Hopping once again lead the team and looked at the seizure chart.

"The Phenytoin has unfortunately given her significant ataxia. This will wear off over the next day or two. I think you should put her in a wheelchair if you leave the room, just till her balance improves. Her lip doesn't need any stitches and her teeth are all intact. I will fill in an ACC form though just in case anything happens down the track with them. I should have time to look over the video EEG today, properly. I had a quick look yesterday and there's a lot of movement artefact, unfortunately, but I'll take a good look and let you know what it shows. I have the MRI appointment for Mikayla tomorrow at nine thirty, so an orderly will collect her before that. We'll stop the Phenytoin tonight, and I'd like to try some Lorazepam, just to try and get some reprieve. Lorazepam can't be given regularly, but hopefully it will help to slow things down for her, okay?"

"Okay, thank you," we said.

The doctors all left and the nurses brought in a wheelchair for Mikayla to use if we needed it. "It's a gorgeous day outside today," she said. "Feel free to take a stroll outside in the wheelchair. Ronald McDonald house have a room for you to use from tonight too. It's the one not on the hospital ground though. It's in Grafton Mews, just a short walk down the road. Do you know where it is?"

"Yes, we saw the signs for it. Thanks so much," Dave said.

"Right. Well I'll go and get Mikayla's medications, and anything else you need just say. There's parking down there too so you could put your car down there, it's free, save paying in the main carpark."

"Great thanks," he said.

She left and we made our morning calls to our parents and texted work and friends. Dave made some work calls and came back in the room with hot drinks for us. "Kylie, I'm going to have to go back to Tauranga tomorrow....those people want to put an offer on that house they looked at last weekend, and

I really don't want to miss out on income….I could come back in a day or two…"

"Okay," I said thinking. "Mum and Dad said if we needed anything just to say. I'll see if they can come up and help us. We have that room now so they can sleep there and we can swap over like we've been doing. I'll give them a ring."

Mum and Dad were fine to come up. They planned to come up tomorrow morning.

Dave took our things, got the car and went down to the Ronald McDonald House in Grafton Mews to book us in. He was shown round and gave them our names and my parents' names explaining what would be happening tomorrow. It was a truly humbling experience looking round the House. So many families from out of the Auckland area with sick children. He couldn't get over the food donations, care and love from strangers under one roof. It was the closest I had seen my husband to tears when he came back. "It's just amazing the generosity people are showing down there," he said. "People volunteering their time to helping others. It's amazing! It's a beautiful place. It really is. Let's head out after lunch and I can show you and Mikayla around it too."

"Okay. Hayden and Teresa are going to pop in again too later. He rung me when you were out."

"Great. Will be nice to get some fresh air."

After lunch, which Mikayla had to eat carefully with her sore mouth, we bundled her up and put her in the wheelchair we had been given to use. Hayden and the family turned up and we all left for a nice walk in the sun. It was so lovely to be outside. You so appreciate the little things when nothing is normal. Feeling the sun and air on us was magic. Hayden pushed the wheel chair and we walked all around the hospital grounds. Then we went down to Ronald McDonald House and Dave showed us our room and how the kitchen ran. We had our own fridge and freezer compartment in a large row of appliances. We also had a labelled shelf in the pantry. There was also an area with shared food which had either been left by previous families, or were donated. Everything was spotless, and the people I saw were happy and friendly, even though I knew everyone had their own hard story of why they were there.

Then we left and carried on to walk round the Auckland museum and gardens. It was a long walk, but just what we all needed. We said goodbye to Hayden, Teresa and the children at the door going back into Starship, and I promised to keep them updated on Mikayla. She looked so much better when Dave lifted her back into her bed. Still pale but with pink cheeks from the fresh air.

That evening we got Mikayla sorted as usual and the nurse brought in her medications.

"So this is one milligram of lorazepam," she said. "Plus her usual meds, the Epilim and Tegretol. Here's your seizure chart too."

"Great, thanks. Well, I'm going to go down to Ronald McDonald House for a sleep now honey." I bent to kiss Mikayla. "See you a bit later."

"Bye Mummy." Although she was still unsteady on her feet her nausea had completely stopped and her speech was back to normal.

I left and enjoyed the short walk down to the room. Dave had told me to order a taxi to bring me back to the hospital later as it would be dark and unsafe to walk back alone. It was lovely to have a bath that night, I even put in some bubbles. Then I snuggled into the comfortable bed and had the best sleep ever. I had set my alarm for two o'clock and got up and dressed when it went off. I brushed my teeth and hair and rung for a taxi to meet me out the front. The security guard at the house wasn't surprised to see me. He said parents often go to see their children at the hospital at all hours of the night. The taxi arrived and took me to Starship. I apologised as it was such a short drive, but he said it was fine and better to use him than walk alone in the dark. They said as it was a quiet night that they would wait for Dave to take him back to the house. I thanked the taxi driver and entered the building. It was more difficult to get back into the hospital. As it was night there was security everywhere. They checked on a large manifold that indeed Mikayla was a patient in the hospital and in the ward I told them. Another guard rung forward to let the nurses know I was coming. It was very thorough.

Finally, I got to Mikayla's room and saw Dave. "How's she?" I asked.

"Much better tonight, she's had ten so far. She's still a bit wobbly, so keep an arm on her when she has one. The nurse said the lorazepam can make you a bit wobbly too."

"That's great she's getting a better sleep," I said. "Now go and have a good sleep. Don't hurry back in the morning. We're going for the MRI about nine o'clock. Mum and Dad hope to be here about ten. The taxi is waiting down below to take you to Ronald McDonald House."

"Okay, better go then, see you in the morning," he hugged me and left.

The rest of the night went well. She was quite wobbly on her legs, but only had a further nine seizures.

By morning she had had nineteen, but I let her wake naturally rather than making her stay awake.

"Bit better night," the nurse smiled as she came in to do Mikayla's obs. "Still busy, but a bit better. How's your lip feel Mikayla?"

"Bit sore when I eat, but it's okay," she said. Her lip was swollen but the cut looked much better this morning.

"Well, we'll get you some breakfast and be ready for the orderly to take you down to MRI at nine, okay?" We both nodded.

"Great, well, obs look good. The doctors will probably catch up with you when you back from your MRI."

At nine o'clock Mikayla was wheeled down to MRI. I actually knew the girl doing the scan. She was in my class at university. "Hi Karen," I said.

"Kylie, how are you?" she asked as she gave me a hug.

"Better today," I told her. "This is Mikayla, Mikayla this is Karen."

"Hi," she said.

Mikayla was very good during the MRI, and after half an hour it was done.

"Those results should be up in the ward in a few hours," Karen said.

"Thanks so much."

Back in the ward we found Dave. "How did you sleep?" I asked him.

"Amazing! Comfiest bed ever! Here's the key," he said handing it to me. "I've packed my things and they're in the car."

"Well you go whenever you need. Mum and Dad should be here soon."

"I'm meeting the clients at three o'clock so I'll leave soon. No hurry."

My Mum and Dad arrived later that morning. "How's our girl?" Mum asked hugging Mikayla.

"I'm good. There's a cool playroom here Nana," said Mikayla.

"Wonderful. You can show us very soon." She smiled to Mikayla. "How are you two?" Mum asked.

"It's been pretty rough," Dave said. "The lorazepam last night probably halved the seizures. She's still a bit wobbly from the Phenytoin from the night before. That didn't do anything."

"It's quite a juggling act isn't it," said Dad.

The doctors came in from doing their rounds and I introduced my parents.

"Hi," said Dr Hopping. "Well, I've looked at the video EEG and I'd say the seizures are happening very deep within the frontal lobe. There's only a very subtle change seen on the waveforms. I've had to convince my colleagues what I'm seeing, but I can see it. So, I do believe we're dealing with intractable frontal lobe seizures, which are mainly nocturnal. Intractable meaning that they are difficult to manage with medications. In saying that, the lorazepam has helped a little I see," she said looking at the seizure chart. "I think we keep that up again tonight, and I'd like to try another medication called Topiramate."

"What are its side effects?" I asked.

"Well, drowsiness, dizziness, coordination problems…"

"Similar to most then," I said. As with all anti-epileptic drugs there are many possible side effects, but to find one that might stop, or even minimise the amount of seizures, was worth the risks.

"I see you had the MRI this morning too. We should get those results later today. How's your mouth today Mikayla?"

"Okay," said Mikayla and Dr Hopping had a look up close at it.

We thanked the doctors and they left to continue their rounds.

"She's a lovely lady. So young," said Mum.

"She's amazing and so good. Her knowledge is incredible. It's really reassuring."

After a cup of tea Dave decided to get on the road. It was a three hour drive back to Tauranga and he had to be back for the appointment.

"I'll give you a ring tonight, early," he said hugging me. He hugged Mikayla. "You look after everyone Mikayla," he joked with her. She gave him a grin and off he went.

We decided to go for a walk down to the Ronald McDonald House after lunch so I could show Mum and Dad around. Mikayla was still a little wobbly so we took her in the wheelchair. Mum and Dad were most impressed with the House, as we were, and I told Dad he should park their car down there and walk up the road to save on parking fares.

"Have to see how your mother's legs go, going up that hill," he joked.

When we got back to the room in Starship the nurse said the results of the MRI were normal. A tiny bit of movement, but nothing obviously abnormal on the scan.

"Well, that's good," I said.

That night the nurses brought in the Topiramate medication with the Tegretol, Epilim and the Lorazepam. It was a few pills for her to swallow, but she managed fine as usual. I got Mikayla all ready for bed and said thank you and goodbye to Mum and Dad. I was going down to the House for a sleep first.

"Take as long as you need Kylie," said Dad.

"Okay, thanks. I'll see if the taxi can wait for you both to take you down to the House when I come up too. Will depend how busy they are."

"Okay." I hugged my parents and Mikayla and walked down to the House. I rung Dave before I went to sleep and updated him on the afternoon and to see how the appointment went.

"It's looking good, hopefully I'll have a contract together tomorrow."

"That's wonderful, well done honey," I said.

We said goodnight and I had a wonderful sleep. I'd set the alarm for three o'clock and when it went off I dressed and tidied up for my parents to stay. I rung for a taxi and went out to meet it. The security guard recognised me from the night before and we exchanged a smile. The taxi was happy to wait for my parents, and I hurried through the hospital to relieve them. When I finally got to Mikayla's door Mum and Dad were both reading books and looked up when I opened the door. They each gave me a big smile. "She's had none!" my Mum quickly rushed to tell me.

"What! None?! That's amazing!" It was honestly the most incredible news. The feeling of relief was huge.

I looked at the seizure chart just to ensure I was hearing it right and smiled at them. "Thank goodness," I said hugging them.

"She got up to go to the toilet just after midnight. That's it. She's walking normally now too," said Mum.

"Wonderful! Just all so good!" I smiled. "Now the taxi is waiting for you guys so you'd better go. Have a lovely sleep and we'll see you in the morning. Don't hurry. Thank you so much." I hugged them again and they left.

I sat on the parents' bed and was just so happy. I googled Topiramate on my phone and read all about it. This was the medication that was going to work, I really hoped so anyway.

Mikayla slept all night! I couldn't wait to ring Dave in the morning and his parents to update them both. I spoke to Aleisha she said, "So you can come home now?"

"Soon baby, soon. I can't wait to see you."

The doctors did their rounds and were very happy to see Mikayla had had no seizures, and was looking alert, and walking and talking normally.

"I'd like to see how tonight goes, and I'd like to reduce the Tegretol by half, keep the Epilim dose the same, and the Topiramate and Lorazepam. If tonight is good you can look to go home. I'll organise a plan though which Dr Downing can manage for you in Tauranga, so let him know if you have any seizure breakthroughs. I'd like to slowly increase the Topiramate over the next fortnight and reduce the

Tegretol till she's off it. She can't be on Lorazepam regularly as it will become ineffective, so over the next few days we'll use it then we'll try and stop it and see how she goes just with the increased Topiramate. So see how tonight goes and we'll go from there." We thanked the doctors and they left.

"Well, that all sounds good," said Mum. "Hopefully this new medicine will keep working."

"Yes, hopefully," I said. We had seen this initial positive effect before with both the Tegretol and the Clobazam so I hoped this wouldn't follow suit.

We filled in the day with walks and the playroom, and I updated Dave and Lyn on what the Doctors said.

"If we do get discharged tomorrow Mum and Dad could take me and Mikayla home. We could meet you at the bottom of the Kaimais or something," I said.

"Sounds good. Just keep me informed."

I didn't tell Aleisha we were definitely coming home tomorrow just in case we didn't as she would be disappointed, but I did tell Lyn there was a possibility.

That night we got Mikayla ready for bed and she had her medications from the nurse. I said goodnight and went down to the House for my sleep. I set my alarm and snuggled down for a sleep hoping that up at the hospital they were having a good night. When I arrived there just before three o'clock I was greeted once again by smiles from my parents. "None again!" they beamed.

"That's wonderful!" I agreed. We said goodbye and Mum and Dad went down to meet the taxi to take them to the House.

Mikayla woke at seven o'clock with a big stretch. "Hi baby," I hugged her. "None again!"

We were both so happy and so was the nurse when she came in to take Mikayla's obs. "Wonderful news!" she said. "Dr Hopping will be happy."

When I went down to make a cup of coffee leaving Mikayla watching morning television, I noticed Christmas decorations had been put up in the corridor. Time had passed without me actually realising it was December the first today. Christmas was just around the corner. We would be home soon and could get back to some normality for Christmas, and I found myself smiling and hoping this positive feeling would stay.

When Dr Hopping came to see us on her rounds she was very pleased to hear Mikayla had had no seizures.

"Its great news, very pleasing. So I can see no reason to keep you here. Please contact Dr Downing if anything changes or you have any concerns. He can get in contact with me if he needs to. We'll write up a sheet for you to follow to slowly increase the Topiramate and decrease the Tegretol and Lorazepam. I would eventually like the Lorazepam just to be given if she is having seizures rather than given every night with her regular meds. I would like to see Mikayla here in one of my clinics in about six weeks' time too if that's okay. Just to check things are still on track. We'll contact you with an appointment time." Then she examined Mikayla and said all looked fine and we could leave.

"Thank you so much Dr Hopping," I said and I thanked her team also.

"Well, we can go home darling," I said to Mikayla. I text Mum and Dad in case they were still asleep to tell him the news and told them to pack up everything at the House and check us out. I told them the plan to meet Dave at the bottom of the Kaimais if that was okay too. Then I rung Dave to tell him the good news and said I'd text when we had a time to meet later that day at the bottom of the Kaimais. I rung Lyn and Colin to give them the good news. Aleisha was so excited to hear we were coming home and seeing her again. She was going back to our house with Dave anyway that day but now she would have us all at home with her.

"We can put up the Christmas tree this weekend too sweetheart," I told her. She was very excited and we hung up looking forward to seeing each other later today.

Mum and Dad walked in about half an hour later and I told them what Dr Hopping had said. "Wonderful news," said Mum.

"I just need to get the prescription filled down at the chemist for her medications then we can go," I said.

Half an hour later we had everything packed and we were ready to go. The nurse gave us our discharge paperwork and we were on our way. We thanked everyone for all their care and help. It's a strange feeling leaving hospital after being so scared and unwell. I can only imagine how it must be to be here for months or even longer. The staff become like family, going through all the ups and downs with you. It's a truly special hospital, that's for sure.

We met Dave at the designated place and thanked Mum and Dad for everything they'd done for us, and said goodbye. We continued on home.

Lyn met us at home with Aleisha. We thanked her so much for looking after Aleisha and after a cup of tea with us she left.

It was lovely to be home again and see Aleisha and the boys. We put up the Christmas tree that weekend and got back to normal family life. We planned for me to go back to work on Monday, and the girls to school.

Chapter Eleven

Mikayla did well for the next month. Her seizures were very minimal and she still had a lot of nights with none. I noticed she was quite tired, and it was difficult to get her out of bed for school in the morning, but I thought she was probably just catching up on all the lost sleep she had missed out on while she was unwell. School was finishing up for the year so the school days were fun and light-hearted for her. I was called into school to see the Deputy Principal to discuss Mikayla's schooling. Mrs Richards was a lovely lady who had spoken to me off and on throughout Mikayla's schooling and knew all about her ill health. She had been concerned back in Year Four that Mikayla was not reaching the standards she should've been due to not being able to retain things. We felt this was due to tiredness from seizures all night and possibly the medications she was on. Now, here was Mikayla at the end of Year Five and I was here again.

"Unfortunately she's quite behind now Kylie," she told me. "In recent testing her cognition testing has been extremely worrying. We asked the children to read this paragraph and answer the questions pertaining to the text, but Mikayla was not able to do this at all. We ended up going backwards and she really only comprehended the text at a Year Three level. I'm also concerned about her maths knowledge. It's difficult for her to retain knowledge and this is obvious in Maths. So....it's very hard for me to say this, but I would like to retain Mikayla in Year Five for next year. It's not a decision we take lightly and I've spoken of Mikayla regularly with Mr Sutton, the principal, and he also feels we need to solidify things with Mikayla next year and help her get ready for Intermediate. She's just going to flounder if we continue her to Year Six next year. What are your thoughts?"

"Well….it's actually a relief to hear you say this," I told her. "We've been concerned too, but actually getting through each night and getting through these bad times has been paramount….so her schooling was second. But yes. To repeat Year Five would be good. She's so little too, I don't think it would be noticeable that she's older than the other children, and hopefully we can use next year to fill in some gaps in her learning."

"Wonderful. Glad you agree…..the other thing is I'd like to try and get funding through for Mikayla to have a teacher aide. It probably would only be a few hours a day but hopefully it would help her too. Now, the red tape is long and there's lots of paperwork. I have a lady I use to help do the applications, so if it's okay with you I'd like to tell her all about Mikayla and she can get the ball rolling…"

"Sounds wonderful. Yes any help we can get her would be great," I said.

That evening we sat Mikayla down and told her about Mrs Richards' conversation.

"So, it means you would have another two years at primary school before Intermediate to try and learn all the things you've missed because you've been too tired okay?" I said.

"So I won't go to Intermediate with Megan and Connor?" she asked.

"No. But when you do get there they'll be there already and can show you around…and you'll have new friends too, children you don't even know yet."

"Okay," she said. As usual Mikayla took it all in her stride. Luckily for us this decision didn't worry her much at all.

We had a lovely Christmas at our place with Dave's family and my parents. It felt like things were all going well and we looked forward to our regular camping holiday and a better year ahead.

When we were camping at the camping ground in Ohope I noticed Mikayla getting more and more lethargic. She was having sleeps during the day, every day for at least two hours. I would put a mattress in our gazebo and stay at our site with her reading my book while she slept. It was concerning, but I thought she had a bit of a virus as she was also not very hungry, and was gagging quite often when she ate. Her seizures were still fairly well controlled just a few every other night. One night I had both the girls asleep in the tent while I sat outside having a wine with Dave. We heard a strange sound inside the tent and thought it was Mikayla having a seizure but it was Aleisha. She was lying on her side in bed her body convulsing, her eyes were rolled back and her face was contorted. She was dribbling from her mouth. I sat beside her to comfort her. I was upset as she had gone so many months without a seizure I was hoping we were in the clear with her. Unfortunately the seizure just went on and on. She had been seizing over five minutes and Dave said we should ring the ambulance. This scared me more as to call the ambulance seemed scary, and how long would they take to get to us at the campground, it was a fifteen minute drive to us from Whakatane. I rung 111, the emergency number, for the first time in my life and shook as I told the operator what was happening and where we were. She said an ambulance was on the way and wouldn't be long as they had just finished a job in Ohope. She asked could someone be at the entrance to the camp ground to show them where our tent was. Then Aleisha began to stop seizing. The convulsions began to slow and her eyes returned to normal looking. I relayed this to the operator who said the paramedic should still look her over as it was a long seizure. I thanked her and hung up. Dave stayed with Aleisha and I ran through the camp ground towards the entrance. On the way I ran into Ryan and quickly told him what had happened. I asked him if he could direct the ambulance to our tent when it arrived. He took off to meet the ambulance and I returned to the tent. Aleisha was trying to speak to Dave and her voice was slurring badly.

"We're here darling, don't talk just rest," I told her stroking her forehead. The ambulance pulled up outside our tent within five minutes and a paramedic hopped out with his medical bag.

"Hello everyone. How is she now?" he asked.

"She's stopped seizing about five minutes ago, thank goodness. She's in here," Dave told him, showing him where Aleisha was. By now Mikayla was awake and confused with what was happening. I told her Aleisha had had a seizure.

"Why is the ambulance man here?" she asked.

"It was a very long seizure," I told her.

The paramedic examined Aleisha and also did a finger prick to check her blood sugar levels which she wasn't happy having done and started to cry.

"Everything looks fine," he told us standing up off the floor of the tent. "If you have any further concerns please call us again. But she looks fine now."

"Thank you so much," Dave said showing him out.

"Right girls, back to sleep then," I said settling them back into their sleeping bags. Aleisha was fine the rest of the night.

We spoke of the night the next morning and couldn't believe we'd had to call the ambulance. We hoped that would be the last time we'd have to do that.

The rest of the holiday Aleisha was fine, but Mikayla continued to be off her food and terribly lethargic, especially in the afternoons. She would sleep each day for a few hours in the gazebo. It was very worrying, but we thought she had a virus and would come right.

The rest of the school holidays flew by and school began again before we knew it.

Aleisha was in Year Four and Mikayla repeating Year Five. Both girls were excited to go back to school and see their friends again. Aleisha seemed fine. She had had no seizures since the one in the tent, and when I had contacted Dr Downing about it he had said to leave her Epilim level the same, as it was just one seizure and she hadn't had one in so long. He hoped it was just from being overtired from the holiday or something similar. So, she was still on the ten milligrams of liquid Epilim morning and night. Mikayla, however was not doing so well. I noticed she was losing weight quickly and her appetite was diminished. She looked pale and was very lethargic and even her hair seemed to be limp and falling out more when I brushed it. When I told Dr Downing he told me to reduce her Topiramate dose slightly to see if that helped so I did.

Over the next few months her seizures slowly increased again in number and decreasing the Topiramate dose hadn't helped with her weight loss and lethargy. Her school teacher, Miss Forbes, whom I was in almost daily contact with, said she was so tired at school she slept every afternoon now, on a beanbag in the back of the classroom. Of course this was upsetting. Mikayla was meant to be 'filling in the gaps' this year and instead she was asleep every afternoon. Unfortunately, because Mikayla was asleep, she was also having seizures at school. At first she was taken to the office when this occurred and Dave or I was rung to collect her. But as this was occurring daily, the school said if it was okay with us they would look after her at school. This was totally going the extra mile for us, as it was difficult for Miss

Forbes who had to keep an ear out for Mikayla in the back of her class having a sleep, and possibly a seizure, at any stage, while teaching the other children. It meant that Dave and I didn't get rung nearly every day to collect her too which had been cutting into our work days. The other children in the class were amazing. The acceptance the children had for Mikayla seizing in the classroom was incredible. They never laughed at her or teased her. As one child told Miss Forbes, 'Mikayla can't help it. She was born with it.' Mikayla had some lovely friends who looked out for her and helped her with her schoolwork she had missed while she was asleep.

The paperwork to get a teacher aide was still being done. It was a long process, and as Mikayla was asleep most afternoons for an hour or so, Miss Forbes did as much as she could with her in the mornings. I kept in contact with Dr Downing so he knew how Mikayla was. I wasn't sure if her tiredness was caused from the seizures or her medication, but it was getting extreme, and I was worried. I weighed Mikayla and couldn't believe it. I knew she had lost weight by looking at her, but the scales said she had lost two and a half kilos since being in Starship in November. Dr Downing called us in for an appointment. He had been speaking to Dr Hopping from Starship and they decided to decrease the Topiramate some more and spoke of beginning Lamotrigine, a new drug. They also wanted a repeat MRI scan as there was slight movement on the one done at Starship. Any focus area which may be causing the seizures would be tiny so the scan needed to be totally still to show this. As Tauranga now had a 3T scanner like Starship, it was organised to be done here.

The doctors also spoke of a Genetic Epilepsy Research Group which was part of the University of Otago, and that they would like the girls to be enrolled with it. They were fairly sure that the girls' epilepsy was caused by genetics, and to be part of the research group may prove beneficial in the future, so we agreed to go into the study.

Dave and I were managing the best we could. I would go to bed early and sleep till two o'clock and Dave would sit up and attend to Mikayla by himself till then. I would have to wear earplugs so that Mikayla didn't wake me, and even then I still heard her most of the time. Then at two o'clock Dave would come to bed and I would look after her till morning. We were both so tired and struggling to get through the day if we were at work. My boss had brought me aside and asked if there was anything they could do to help. Did I want to drop a day perhaps? But money was tight and we needed all the days I could manage as Dave was finding it difficult to get deals together being so tired also.

Both our sets of parents were doing all they could. Lyn and Colin had the girls often in the weekends so we could get sleep. In the end we asked my parents to come over and stay Sunday nights while we slept at Lyn and Colin's. Mum and Dad got the girls to school and we went to work. Then we chose a night during the week to drop the girls at Lyn and Colin's so we could go to work refreshed. It was a great help but it felt like we were barely getting through, just going through the paces, but not really living.

Mikayla's medications now were Epilim, Topiramate and Lorazepam, if we needed to use it during the night. We found that the one milligram dose wasn't doing anything though, so Dr Downing increased it to a two-point-five milligram tablet, with instructions to give half if needed, and if no reduction in seizures in the next forty five minutes, to give the other half. On nights where we had given Mikayla a whole two-point-five milligram tablet, she was so tired in the morning we could hardly get her out of bed for school. Her legs were wobbly and she had no energy. It was so hard to know what to do. Do one of us call in sick from work and keep her home.....or do we send her to school and they'll ring us in an hour because she's too tired. Most days were the same and she wasn't learning anything. So much for repeating the year to fill in what she'd missed. The poor kid was just so tired and showing more and more weight loss. It was so hard to see her like that.

I remember one day dropping her at school as close as I could get to the school entrance. I looked in the rear vision mirror as I drove away, and I got tears in my eyes. This tiny child with her school bag which now looked too big for her back, walking so slowly into school it was taking all her effort to put one foot in front of the other. I felt torn, so mean for sending her to school, so tired myself, and needing to go to work as my own sick leave was very low from all the time I'd been in hospital with Mikayla. Dave had so much time off with Mikayla his business was suffering badly which was adding stress to our marriage. Extreme tiredness, with now financial worries, and worries about Mikayla were putting us all at our breaking points.

I confided in my friend, Melissa, "Surely you can get respite care," she told me. "Another friend I know gets it and they get more sleep than you do."

I was desperate for help and rung our Medical Centre to tell the nurse about what was happening. She said she'd make some calls and someone would contact me. By the end of the day a lady rung me from Support Net.

"Hi, I'm Georgia. When can I come and see you?" she asked. We arranged a time for the following day. Georgia took notes as I explained our situation to her. I told of how Dave and I do 'shifts' through the night. Dave staying awake till two o'clock and then I take over to look after Mikayla till morning. I told her how we can only stop the seizures by keeping her awake and using lorazepam, but that the lorazepam makes it hard to get her up in the mornings to go to school. I told her that Dave and I had missed a lot of work too, due to either being too tired, or having to stay home with Mikayla.

"Gosh, it's certainly been hard for you all. I'm sorry you haven't had help before now," she said. She explained that she would now try and get funding for Mikayla to have in-home respite care.

"The money is held with a company and they pay the carers. You need to ring around and try and find carers to help you. Here's a list of some agencies that may be able to help," she said handing me a sheet of paper.

She rung me later that day with the amount of money that Mikayla had for carers. It equated to two nights of care at night that we could get. I rung all the agencies and more from the telephone book. Most were not keen on the type of work or the hours involved. A lot cared for the elderly and weren't keen on looking after an epileptic child. Most wanted a bedroom for the carer and a lot costed more than we had allocated for in our funding. Finally, when I thought it wasn't going to work, I came across an agency who said they would make it work. When I told them our story I think the owner felt sorry for us. She said she had two ladies who could work. They would visit us in the next few days to meet Mikayla and see what was involved. I was so thankful and relieved and couldn't wait to tell Dave that we had some permanent help coming. It was like having two angels coming to the rescue. Two nights where we could try and sleep, and someone else would attend to Mikayla's seizures. After years of sleepless nights it was amazing. We had to get earplugs and try to block out Mikayla's seizures which we were so used to getting up to. But for those two nights we tried to rest and they could get us if they needed to.

Mikayla's weight continued to drop off her. We saw Dr Downing again and he prescribed Fortisip drinks for Mikayla to try and get some weight on her. I begged Mikayla to drink them but she just couldn't drink them. We tried all three flavours and nothing appealed to her. The taste and the amount of liquid was just too much for her. She ended up gagging each time.

Her teacher aide was finally sorted and started in June, six months after first trying to get help. Mikayla had twelve hours of teacher aide help. The hours were meant to be used for the care of Mikayla while in school. So while she slept they were to watch over her and look after her while she had a seizure, rather than actually helping her academically. I found this frustrating, but considering how sick she was and how little learning she was actually doing, it was where the need was at present anyway.

One day Mikayla was in the bath when she called out to me. She was so tired she didn't have to energy to get out. I went to her and as she stood up in the bath I had to hold in my gasp. She was tiny. Absolutely scarily bony. Her ribs and hip bones stood out from her skin. Her tiny body looked so malnourished I was in shock. Her long hair hung limp and thin, so much was falling out when I brushed it. I helped her dry and dress and put her to bed. I told Dave, "She's even thinner than we thought. She's got to see someone this is bad."

Chapter Twelve

Two days later Mikayla had her MRI scan. It was a very scary day. I took her to the scanner and my friends and colleagues were there. They called us through to get changed and couldn't believe how small Mikayla had got. During the scan Mikayla closed her eyes and slept. I was worried she might jump up and have a seizure and hurt herself but we were okay. Afterwards Dr Dunn, my friend and Radiologist who always asked about the girls, pulled me aside.

"Kylie, unfortunately, comparing all three of her MRIs, todays shows some parenchymal volume loss. Let me show you." He pointed out some areas on today's scan.

"Is that caused from all the seizures?" I asked.

"I don't think so," he said, "I think its weight loss…. she really needs some help Kylie and I think you need to take her into hospital. She needs to see a Dietician and needs a nasogastric tube. It's the only way you'll be able to get some weight on her now and you mustn't leave without it, okay."

"Okay I said." I had tears in my eyes. I couldn't believe her weight had gotten this bad. My little girl was fading away before my eyes.

Dr Dunn wished us well and my boss who was part of the team doing Mikayla's scan told me to take as much time off as I needed. "You have to take her today Kylie, don't worry about work…." I thanked her and took Mikayla to get redressed in her clothes. I went home and packed a bag and rung Dave and told him what I had been told and the MRI scan result. Then I took Mikayla to A and E. They were busy and it took ages to get called through, then I had to tell each doctor I saw about Mikayla's seizures, weight loss, and MRI result. They all said, "How many seizures?!" and I would say, "there's nothing you can do about that, but I'm worried about her weight loss…" We finally got sent to the Children's Ward. The Paediatrician we saw was lovely, but after an hour talking was going to send us home. I asked, "Could we please see a dietician?" and after an hour Kelly Michaels introduced herself to us.

She was efficient and friendly, and listened closely to our whole story. My voice was shaking by the end, I was almost begging this woman to help us. Kelly said, "Mikayla needs a naso-gastric tube. There's no way she's going to put weight on without it. You'll be here for at least a few days while we try and get some weight on her. She needs a blood test. We need to check her kidneys and her blood levels. Okay?"

"Yes," I breathed. "Thank you."

It was such a relief. Kelly weighed Mikayla and I was shocked. She was twenty-one-point-two kilograms. She had lost three and a half kilos since being in Starship in November.

A nurse took Mikayla into a treatment room with a jungle theme painted on one of the walls. She explained to us what inserting a nasogastric tube involved, and what Mikayla needed to do. She measured what size tube Mikayla would need and opened some gloves and the tube from their packets. I held Mikayla's hand as she lay on the bed, her head propped up on pillows. The nurse slowly inserted the tube into Mikayla's nostril, and pushed it gently in and down. Mikayla didn't like it and cried out a little. "Swallow now," the nurse instructed. "Swallow," I repeated, holding Mikayla's hand and begging her to do it. It wasn't pleasant for Mikayla, but in just a minute the tube was in position. The nurse taped the tube, wrapping the tape to Mikayla's nostril. She took a small strip of litmus paper from a canister and a syringe which she connected to the end of the nasogastric tube. She drew back on the syringe till some fluid filled it. She unscrewed the syringe and put a little fluid on the litmus paper which she showed me matched the acidic level on the canister meaning the end of the tube was in the correct place, being in Mikayla's stomach. This was the procedure I was to follow when I did her feeds at home. If the tube was not in her stomach correctly it would be dangerous to start the feed. The phlebotomist came in not long after and did her blood test.

Back in our room the nurse showed me how to do Mikayla's feeds through her nasogastric tube. We were starting with very small amounts of fluid, and for the first feed she had twenty milligrams of the fluid feed going through the tube using gravity to get it through. She held the syringe high above Mikayla's head and the feed dripped through her nose. The first time she hated it. It felt strange coming through the tube and the coldness of the fluid felt strange down her nose and throat. I don't know if it was the strange feeling, or whether her stomach had shrunk, but with less than the twenty milligrams in her stomach she began to throw up. It wasn't pleasant and the nurse told me we really don't want her to throw up as it can also dislodge the tube.

Over the day Mikayla got used to the tube feeds and stopped vomiting. By the next day I was doing the feeds by myself and the nurse popped in now and then to watch. Mikayla's blood test came back with a very low phosphate level. We were told this happened sometimes with malnutrition from lack of food. They started her on a medication to try and raise the phosphate level. We stayed in hospital for four days and slowly, even in this short space of time, Mikayla put on half a kilogram. She was continuing eating as normal, and we topped up her meals with the feeds through the nasogastric tube three times a day. When we left the hospital Mikayla's Phosphate level was back to normal so she could stop that medication. Kelly came to see us before we were discharged and gave us her card if I had any problems once we were home. She also gave us some liquid feed for Mikayla. I thanked her for all her help. If we hadn't seen Kelly I think Mikayla could've got into real trouble.

At home we managed the feeds well. We got up a bit earlier in the mornings to get the breakfast feed done before school and work. Mikayla was still having seizures as usual so some mornings were tricky to get her up to get it all done. I had told the girls' school that they might be slightly late some mornings due to the nasogastric feed. We got the time taken to do the feed shortened by starting to slowly push the liquid down the tube using the plunger as she was tolerating it more now. She absolutely loved the feeling of fullness in her tummy from the additional food and she was putting on weight steadily. Either Dave or I would go into school at lunchtime to do her lunch feed. The school kindly gave us the old dental clinic to use to do her feeds as it had a sink for cleaning up too. Mikayla must've really liked the energy and fullness the feeds gave her because she would ask for just a little more when we'd finish, but sometimes that extra bit would make her vomit. Five times she dislodged her nasogastric tube. It would end up half out her mouth and the other end out her nose. I would have to pull it out and take her into hospital to get another tube put down. She was such a trouper because it can't have been pleasant.

Dr Downing gave us a letter which gave Mikayla direct admission to the children's ward to get her tube reinserted if it came out and also if her seizures got uncontrollable. This was wonderful because having to go through A and E each time was very tedious having to explain the same thing over and over again to each doctor. After six weeks Mikayla had put on three kilograms and was looking so much better. She was still small, but she had more energy and had lost the real gaunt look she had before.

We saw Dr Hopping a few weeks later in a clinic in Tauranga. She didn't like all that had happened with Mikayla's weight loss, lethargy and loss of cognition. She was not doing that well with her seizure control or her schooling. We were told that Mikayla had had the large weight-loss due to a side effect from the Topiramate so it would need to be weaned off again.

"I'd like to start Mikayla on Lamotrigine," she told us. "It will take quite some time to get her up to a level which would offer seizure control, but unfortunately we must do the increases slowly as this medication can cause Stevens - Johnson syndrome if we administer it too quickly. This is a skin rash which can be disfiguring or fatal is not treated. But we've seen wonderful seizure control with this medication so it is worth trying it. This is how you need to do the increases," she told us showing a list of increments on a sheet of paper which we were to follow to bring Mikayla up to fifty milligrams of Lamotrigine in three months' time.

"Will it take this long to see if it will work?" I asked looking over the sheet of paper.

"Hopefully not. I would like to decrease the Epilim dose too when we reach about twenty five milligrams, but keep in touch with Dr Downing and he can let me know how you're going."

"Do you think this one will work?" I asked. I was looking directly at her and could hear the pleading sound to my voice. I just needed to hear something positive.

"I hope so, we need to try it…."

"Yes," I said.

"So decrease the Topiramate like this," she said showing me the decreases on the paper beside the

Lamotrigine increases, "and continue using the Lorazepam if and when required in the night. Continue the Epilim at the current level and we'll look to decrease it slightly when she reaches twenty five milligrams of Lamotrigine."

She examined Mikayla and told us to contact Dr Downing if she lost any weight or had any concerns at all and to be especially aware of any skin rashes as it may be the Stevens - Johnson syndrome. We thanked her and left with all the paperwork.

Mikayla started the Lamotrigine and over the next six weeks she unfortunately got a cold, which seemed to always exacerbate her seizures. We noticed her weight stagnating and her schooling regressing even further. Mikayla now had two teacher aides to help her. The one the school organised for twelve hours of 'care' a week and one through the Northern Health School for two hours a week. Mikayla absolutely loved her Northern Health School teacher aide, Tania, and she was able to come to our house if Mikayla was not at school on her day, and do her lesson at home. It was kept basic as the reason she was home was probably exhaustion from a long night of seizures, but it really brightened her day to see Tania. They got along so well and it was lovely to hear Mikayla giggling to things Tania told her.

We saw Dr Downing for a check-up six weeks after starting the Lamotrigine.

"It's not helping at all so far," Dave told him.

"Yes, I see," he said looking at our seizure record book, "but we have to give it a good try right up to the maximum level for her weight. I see her weight is unchanged since you saw Dr Hopping.”

“Yes and she’s very quiet, not at all bubbly and ‘out there’ like she used to be,” I said.

“We have a cruise ship holiday booked too. Seems silly to go, but we booked it some time ago,” Dave explained. “It’s a week going from Brisbane to Cairns and back. Do you think it will be okay to go?”

“Yes, I can’t see why not,” Dr Downing said. “I’ll write you a letter for the ships’ doctor just outlining Mikayla starting Lamotrigine, and to look out for Stevens-Johnson syndrome and other side effects. Just continue using Lorazepam if needed. It seems to help to stop the seizures effectively isn’t it?”

“Yes it is. We’re using the whole two point five milligrams by the end of the night and she’s very wobbly on her legs and tired in the morning, but it does stop the seizures.”

“Good. Well I’ll get a letter typed up and sent to you. Continue increasing the Lamotrigine. Ring me if you have any concerns, please.” He wrote his cell phone number on a piece of paper and handed it to me. “If you just have a query or are worried about anything. Obviously take her straight to the doctor if it’s serious, but I want to be able to help if you’re worried.”

“Thank you so much,” we both sad. I had tears in my eyes. This man had gone through all this with us and was willing to give us his personal number if we had any worries. “I won’t use it unless we’re really needing it,” I said.

"It's okay," he smiled and showed us out. "Enjoy your holiday."

Chapter Thirteen

The day of our cruise ship holiday arrived, and we drove up to Auckland to stay in the airport hotel as our flight out to Brisbane was very early. We needed to be at the airport at five in the morning. The night before was terrible. Mikayla had a lot of seizures and when the alarm went off at four o'clock we hadn't had a lot of sleep. We packed up and went out the front of the hotel to meet the shuttle to take us to the airport. The girls were very excited and any sleepiness was quickly forgotten. We got to the airport and had breakfast and waited to board our flight to Brisbane. It was only the girls' second time in a plane so it was very exciting as it was a fairly new experience.

We landed in Brisbane and got a taxi to the cruise ship docking area. It was a very long process getting on the ship and by the time we were taken to the docking area we were all exhausted from our early morning start and broken sleeps. Mikayla and Aleisha were both asleep on our laps on the floor and a steward came to us and invited us to board the ship now ahead of the other people. It was lovely of her and we were very grateful.

The photographer wanted a family photo of us as we boarded, and it was not a good photo. Two grumpy girls and two tired adults. We found our room and it was lovely. We had an adjoining room with the girls and a bathroom each. Some cute little animals made out of towels were sitting on our beds which the girls found very amusing. We unpacked and had a quick look round the ship, but we were all a bit tired so decided to go and have a lie down before the compulsory briefing on ship safety everyone had to do out on deck. We all had a wee nap and both the girls were fast asleep when the warning came across the loud speaker to go on deck for the briefing. It was very hard to wake the girls up, they were exhausted.

We lined up on deck with everyone and listened to the safety talk. Afterwards we had a good look around the ship and had a drink on the upper deck watching the ship leave Brisbane harbour. We had a lovely afternoon and evening. The food was great and there was so much variety. We went back to the cabin at seven thirty as the girls were ready for bed.

That night we used a chair to keep the door separating our cabins open so we could attend to Mikayla. She had her usual seizures and we would go through to her cabin to look after her. In the early hours of the morning I awoke to a choking sound and got up expecting to see Mikayla having a seizure, but instead Aleisha was having one. She was convulsing in her bed, her head moving rhythmically to the left and her face contorted. Her eyes were rolled back and she was dribbling. I screamed for Dave and he ran in beside me. The seizure went on and on, and all we could do was stroke her forehead and reassure her. Blood began dripping from her mouth and I couldn't stop crying.

"Her tongue, she's biting her tongue! Dave it's just not stopping!"

"We have to call a doctor," he told me.

"I saw a number in that folder there," I pointed. He found the number in the front of the folder and I picked up the phone and rung it. After one ring I was put through to an operator and I told him what was happening. "I'll get someone to ring you straight away," he told me. I hung up. A minute later the phone rang.

"I'm Sharon, the Ships Nurse, is your daughter still seizing?" she asked.

"Yes, and she's biting her tongue…" I was hiccoughing down the phone. I was terrified, we were in the middle of the ocean and felt very vulnerable.

"Okay, just make sure she stays on the bed and doesn't hurt herself. I'll be right there." She hung up and I told Dave what she had said. Aleisha's seizing then began to slow down. She had her eyes closed but the convulsing stopped. Every few seconds her arm and head would twitch like a bolt of electricity was going through her little body.

"Aleisha, darling it's okay," I told her, "we're here…" There was a knock at the door.

"Come in," Dave said. A woman in her fifties opened the door.

"I'm Sharon," she said. "This must be Aleisha."

"Mummy?" said Mikayla. "What's happening?" she sat up in her bed looking confused.

"Aleisha has had a seizure," I told her. "The nurse is here to see her."

Aleisha just lay there with her eyes closed, having the occasional twitch through her arm and head.

"Why isn't she waking up?" I asked.

"It's the post ictal phase," she told me. "It's common after a long seizure. Aleisha can you hear me?" she said. She took the stethoscope from round her neck and listened to Aleisha's chest. She then took her finger and connected the pulse oximeter probe to it and put a blood pressure cuff round her other arm. "It all looks fine. But I'd like to get her checked over by our ship doctor if that's okay?"

"Yes," we said. "Please do."

I'll just get the wheelchair. It's outside the door," she said, and went outside to get it. "Who's coming with her?" she asked.

"I will," I said looking at Dave. He nodded. Mikayla started to cry.

"She'll be fine, honey," said Sharon to Mikayla. "Just getting her checked over by the doctor. Maybe if you sit in the wheelchair mum, and we'll put Aleisha on your lap," I did as she said and Dave lifted Aleisha from the bed into my lap. She still didn't wake up, it was very scary.

"This is nothing like Mikayla's seizures," I said.

"Oh, you have seizures too?" Sharon asked Mikayla.

"Yes," she snivelled.

"Right, we'll take this blanket. It's a bit cold in the corridors," she said. "Off we go."

"Bye. Won't be long," I said to Dave and Mikayla, who was still looking very upset.

Sharon wheeled us through the ship, down an elevator and into the belly of the ship to the doctors' rooms. Aleisha's eyes opened on the journey and she started to look more awake. In the room a lady was waiting for us.

"Hi, I'm Patricia Kemp, the ships' doctor," she told me. "Your daughter has had a seizure?"

"Yes, this is Aleisha. She's had seizures before, but hasn't had one in ages. We've weaned her off her medication now. She was on Epilim."

"Okay. Hi Aleisha, I'm Doctor Kemp. Can we pop you on the bed here and I'll check everything out. Good girl," she said as I helped her onto the bed. Dr Kemp looked Aleisha all over and found nothing untoward. Her grip was very weak after the seizure and her speech was slurred. Her tongue was all bitten up and was bleeding slightly down one side. She got her some Pamol liquid for the pain and filled out all the paperwork. She told us to contact Dr Downing when we could, but didn't feel Aleisha needed to be put back on Epilim without talking to him first.

"This is her first seizure in a long time. I wouldn't rush to medicate her without speaking to your paediatrician first. We don't have anti-epileptic medication on board anyway, just medications to stop seizures that aren't stopping by themselves."

"Why did she take so long to wake up from the seizure?" I asked.

"It's normal after a grand mal seizure. It's called the post ictal phase. It just takes time for the brain to regain normality after such a traumatic event."

"My other daughter has seizures too but they present so much differently, we just haven't seen that before."

"Okay. Well she looks fine now. Could you pop by tomorrow and I'll check everything is still okay. Contact your paediatrician when you can. Here's my details if he needs to know anything. And please, just ring if you have any further concerns, okay?"

"Thank you," I said.

"Hop back in the chair," Sharon said. "I'll wheel you back. She's still a bit wobbly to walk back."

I did as she said and thanked Dr Kemp again, leaving with the paperwork and Pamol.

We arrived back at our cabin and I knocked for Dave to let us in. He opened the door and I could see Mikayla sitting up in bed doing some drawing.

"She didn't want to go back to sleep," Dave explained.

We thanked Sharon and said goodbye. She closed the door and left with the wheelchair. I told Dave everything the Doctor had said. I hugged him and let out a big sigh.

"I just can't believe it. We're so worried about Mikayla, and then Aleisha has a huge seizure. It's crazy!"

We all tried to get a little more sleep before morning. I text Dr Downing the next morning and he returned my text immediately. He was very sorry to hear about Aleisha's seizure, but agreed with Dr Kemp not to start on any medications as it was her first seizure in such a long time. He felt it had probably come on from extreme tiredness and being so excited.

We continued on with our holiday with no further episodes from Aleisha, and just Mikayla's usual seizures. It certainly wasn't the relaxing holiday we were hoping for, but it was wonderful to experience a cruise ship and we had a great time.

When we got home our friends and family couldn't believe Aleisha had had a seizure on top of all Mikayla's seizures. It certainly wasn't expected.

Over the next month Mikayla reached the maximum level of Lamotrigine for her weight. We had also reduced the Epilim slightly as we'd been told to do. The seizures hadn't reduced at all. The Lamotrigine hadn't helped. Mikayla was also experiencing double vision which wasn't pleasant. She said one day, that my face was 'there…. and there' pointing to two areas around my shoulders. I contacted Dr Downing, who called us in.

"We need to start weaning off the Lamotrigine," he said. "It obviously didn't help with the seizures, and the double vision isn't good either. You won't be able to start anything new till the Lamotrigine level is lower and we need to reduce slowly."

He had contacted Dr Hopping at Starship who had suggested trying Tegretol again so he gave us a script for that. We also asked about other options such as trying acupuncture or essential oils as friends and family had told us about these methods and we were, of course, desperate to find something to help. Dr Downing told us to give them a go. They couldn't do any harm.

Dave had found a company who specialised in oils to help all sorts of ailments, so he contacted them and they advised on using frankincense, so we put it on her forehead and the soles of her feet before bed each night. I'm not sure if it helped that much but her seizures did decrease in frequency slightly, though she had also started the Tegretol again so it may've been that too.

I found a man, Lee, who did acupuncture and I asked him if he'd ever had success in stopping seizures using acupuncture and he said yes. So we began two sessions a week with him. Mikayla fell asleep during every session and I was worried she would have a seizure in the room. Waking her up at the end of each session seemed very cruel as she was sleeping so poorly normally at home. Lee would help me get Mikayla into the car. We tried four months of acupuncture, and it may have helped slightly, but not significantly. What it did help with was her eczema which cleared up a lot and any colds she had at the time. As I said we were desperate to try anything so it was worth a go.

We also looked into Medicinal Cannabis. It was very difficult to obtain and it was a long hard road to get it approved for your child. It was also extremely expensive. We learnt of trials which were underway in adults in Australia and New Zealand for Cannabis gels which were rubbed on the skin. The medicinal properties of the cannabis were in the media everywhere, though we were warned that the negative aspects were often not mentioned, and it wasn't always as positive an outcome as the media showed.

Chapter Fourteen

In October, Mikayla was nearly eleven and had a terrible tummy bug. We had an appointment in Clinic at Starship with Dr Hopping and didn't want to cancel. She had diarrhoea and wasn't eating much at all. I was making her drink water to keep her fluids up. Although she was unwell her seizure control was amazing. We had had no seizures for the last four nights, and put it down to the Lamotrigine being weaned off and the Tegretol working well now even though it was at a very low dose. Dr Hopping examined Mikayla and found her lethargic and tired. Her double vision was only slightly still apparent, so weaning the Lamotrigine was helping here. I was so excited about the Tegretol seeming to stop the seizures, but Dr Hopping said it sounded like a 'honeymoon period' with the Tegretol, as the dose was still way too low to have been helping much.

Sure enough as the days went on Mikayla got better with her tummy bug and the seizures came back with a vengeance. It would be another six months before the real reason for Mikayla's seizures stopping would become apparent.

Over the next three weeks Mikayla's seizures continued to increase in frequency each night, until at the end of October, we used the open admission letter and took Mikayla to Tauranga Hospital again. She was having thirty to forty seizures a night, and Dave and I were absolutely exhausted. Mikayla had missed so much school this term it was sad to admit it, but this catch up year had been a waste of time. She had only been to school for three days so far in the whole term! Apart from those four nights seizure-free when she was unwell, she had had five months of seizures every night.

On the first night being in Hospital the nurses couldn't believe how many seizures she was having. Dave was in with her for the night, and when the nurse came in at seven o'clock for her shift swap, she had tears in her eyes.

"How have you all coped with this at home by yourselves? It's just horrific!" she was very emotional and teary.

"Well, we just have to," said Dave to the nurses, "what else do you do?" Mikayla was sitting up in bed smiling as usual. She was amazing. It was difficult to see how rough a night she had had. "We have carers to help two nights a week. But you can still hear her seizing, and you worry…..it's hard to sleep really."

The Charge Nurse came in that morning when I had come in to swap with Dave. She said to us both that the nurse from that morning had felt we needed some rest, and a carer was being brought in for the nights, so they would look after Mikayla. The nurses were only down the hall if the carer needed any help. There was a spare room down the hall for Dave or I to sleep uninterrupted, so we could get some respite from the sleepless nights. We were so thankful.

"It's the least we can do," said Lauren the Charge Nurse. "Just let me know each morning whether you'll be in for that night, so I can organise care to be there." It was a godsend. I don't think we could've done that part without the help. So we went home, worked each day and one of us would bring Mikayla in each night to be cared for in the hospital, and Dave or I would sleep down the hallway. We both felt alive again after a few nights uninterrupted sleep.

Mikayla however, wasn't having a great time. On the second night she hit her hand so hard on the door during a seizure she needed an x-ray as it was bruised, swollen and sore. The carers were lovely and Mikayla really liked them. The nurses were there if the carers had any worries or problems, and we were just down the hall if needed too. Mikayla's meds were being altered again too by Dr Downing who was liaising with Dr Hopping. The Tegretol was increased further, Clobazam was introduced again as it had helped initially last time it was used, the Epilim was decreased and a new drug was introduced, Lacosamide.

After six nights coming into hospital each night, Dave and I felt much better to continue caring at home. Mikayla's seizures, as usual, each time a new drug was introduced, slowed right down, and we even had some nights seizure-free again. We were optimistic about the Lacosamide. Maybe, this was finally the drug to stop the seizures. But this was short-lived.

After a week the seizures again became frequent. Mikayla had only had a couple more days at school and she was back up to over forty seizures a night. We contacted Dr Downing and he told us Dr Hopping wanted us to go up to Starship. She had booked the Video EEG room again and wanted to start there. We asked Dave's parents, Lyn and Colin, if they would look after Aleisha for us, and Dave and I took Mikayla up to Auckland to Starship.

They took Mikayla into Auckland Hospital to attach the wires to her scalp for the Video EEG. The plan was for her to be monitored on the video EEG for two nights. The first night Mikayla had a staggering sixty two seizures. In the morning she was exhausted. Her hips and shoulders were aching severely from the repetitive seizures. The two point five milligrams of Lorazepam was being given every night by now, and was having minimal effect. Dr Hopping decided to reduce the Lacosamide, as it was not reducing the seizures effectively either. She decided to try steroids to try and stop the seizures. The steroids had a minimal effect the first night.

After two nights of being monitored for the video EEG, Mikayla was moved into another room. Dave had to go back to Tauranga for work, so my mum came up to Starship Hospital by bus from Te Awamutu. We had a room at Ronald McDonald house and we did the shift swaps each night at about two o'clock in the morning, as we did last time we were there.

Dr Hopping also wanted a PET CT Scan and a lumbar puncture to see if anything showed up. Both tests were normal. On the third night Dr Hopping put Mikayla on Acetazolamide, a diuretic. Diuretics were used many years ago to help with seizures. That night Mikayla's seizures reduced, and after two more nights the Acetazolamide completely stopped the seizures. After a total of six nights in hospital we were discharged. Again we were hopeful that this medication would be the one to stop the seizures for good.

Mikayla and I caught a bus back to Tauranga and Mum caught a bus back to Te Awamutu.

The end of 2016 was upon us and the girls finished school for the year. Mikayla had missed most of Term Four, but I was so thankful to her lovely teacher Miss Forbes who had looked after her when she was at school and gone the extra mile for our little girl. I will be forever grateful for her care of Mikayla.

We celebrated Christmas and had our usual camping holiday in Ohope. Both girls' seizures were well controlled. Aleisha having had no seizures since the one on the cruise ship and Mikayla having just the odd night with a few seizures. We were very hopeful for 2017.

Chapter Fifteen

The girls started back at school. Mikayla in Year Six and Aleisha Year Five.

The Acetazolamide worked well for several months with Mikayla having two hundred and fifty milligrams of it morning and night. She was still on Epilim, Clobazam and Tegretol too. Then the seizures started to increase again. They were becoming more combative and aggressive, and were also lasting longer.

By March she was back to having twenty to thirty seizures a night. Mikayla was admitted to Tauranga Hospital. The lorazepam was having minimal effect at breaking the seizures. Mikayla was having to be kept awake during the night to try and break the seizures. We would put her in a wheelchair and walk the wards corridor to try and keep her awake. I met a male nurse one night who told me of meeting parents like us when he worked in a hospital in Sydney years ago.

"They had tried everything," he said. "But childhood epilepsy really is such a difficult thing to treat. Finally they tried medicinal marijuana and it helped immensely."

"Yes, I think it's something to look into," I told him. "I'll talk to our Starship Doctors."

The next day, Dr Downing tried increasing the amount of Acetazolamide, but her blood test showed it was lowering her PH too much, so the Acetazolamide was lowered back down.

The Tegretol was increased and the seizures lowered in frequency again. They were still lasting longer though, and she was more combative than before.

After four nights in hospital Mikayla was discharged.

We had a clinic appointment at Starship in April. We spoke to Dr Hopping about the possibility of starting Mikayla on medicinal cannabis, or getting on a trial, but these options were lengthy and costly, though we were desperate to try something.

At this appointment Dave mentioned that the only time Mikayla's seizures had actually stopped for five or six nights in a row, was when she was extremely unwell with stomach bug or a flu. Dr Hopping found it very interesting that Mikayla's seizures stopped when she was off her food with viruses, and thought it might be an indicator that Mikayla responded well to her body being in a ketosis state, and that the ketogenic diet may help her. This was a difficult path to follow as there was no funding for a dietician to help us in Tauranga, and the diet was extremely strict and difficult to follow for the child and the parents. Dr Hopping suggested trying a low dose of Phenytoin and wrote out a script for this. We also spoke about another medication to try called Zonisamide.

On the drive back home to Tauranga Dave and I spoke non-stop about the next step. We really didn't want to go back on the Phenytoin, even at a low level as this was the drug which caused the ataxia in

Starship when she fell out of bed. We spoke about the discussion we had had about the ketogenic diet.

"I really think we need to look into this. It's surely worth pursuing as ketosis is the only thing that has stopped her seizures," Dave said.

That evening I looked up the ketogenic diet on the internet. There were children on this diet in America who were having amazing results. Their seizures were reducing, and even stopping in some cases. I read that about a third of the children on the diet saw no change, a third saw a fifty percent, or better, reduction in seizures, and a third had their seizures completely stop. It sounded very promising and I thought 'what did we have to lose?' All the sites advised not starting the diet without medical advice, and that the child must be monitored closely by medical personnel. I wrote down the foods which must be avoided and ended up with a list with such foods as potatoes, rice, pasta, flour, bread, sugar, nothing processed, most fruit, and all vegetables which were grown in the ground. I made another list of foods which could be eaten. This list had meats, cheese, Greek yoghurt, eggs, butter, berries, nuts, and low carbohydrate vegetables such as capsicum, celery, courgette, and mushrooms. I read how additional fats needed to be added to the diet to bring the body into ketosis. The body would then burn fat for energy instead of sugar. This fat burning puts the body into ketosis and somehow sedates the brain to minimise the seizures.

We decided to try changing Mikayla's diet. What did we have to lose? We spoke with her about it, and said it was very important that she only ate what we gave her to eat to give this a good try, and she was keen. She was obviously very sick of all the seizures she had had for so many years of her short life, so the thought of reducing, or even stopping these horrible nights, was worth following what we said. Mikayla never had a huge appetite for sweet foods anyway, preferring savoury to sweet. But the thought of no hot chips or roast vegetables was hard for Mikayla. Still, she wanted to give it a go.

We started the next day and cooked her bacon and eggs for breakfast. She went to school with a lunchbox of cold chicken, some blueberries, nuts, dark chocolate and smoked cheese. For dinner we cooked her meat, cabbage, courgette and mushrooms. We contacted Dr Downing to let him know what we had started.

Within ten days Mikayla's seizures had reduced from twenty odd per night, to less than ten!! We were so excited! We knew we were on to something. We had brought a ketone monitoring machine from the chemist. We took a finger prick of Mikayla's blood, and the machine let us know the level of ketones in her blood. This was important as if the ketones levels got too high she would need to get to hospital immediately.

We went to see Dr Downing to talk about the diet more. He said we definitely needed to get some help from a dietician. He was excited to see the results we had achieved already. He told us to write to the head of our District Health Board telling them of Mikayla's story till now, and how we had started the diet and already seen a drop in her seizures.

"Ask for funding for a dietician to help," he said. "Looking at what you're feeding her I think you need more fat and lower carbohydrates, but you need this to be monitored carefully." He advised we write the letter as soon as possible and keep a food diary record for monitoring her daily intake of food. He also wanted a blood test looking at cholesterol, iron, calcium and other nutrients as a baseline, an ECG and an Ultrasound of her kidneys checking for kidney stones which can occur with the extra fats.

We wrote the letter that night and got all the tests done over the next few weeks. Mikayla had an appointment with a dietician even though there was no funding through as yet. Stephanie was lovely and advised us further on Mikayla's diet. She said Mikayla would probably end up on a form of the Modified Atkins diet as the ketogenic diet for epilepsy would be too strict for a child of Mikayla's age. The ketogenic diet requires protein and fluids to also be monitored and weighed out, and this is easier to follow on a younger child.

As Dr Downing had said, we had the carbohydrates too high and the fat intake too low, but we were still seeing some encouraging results. We showed her recipes we had found on the internet and she helped us, showing us what we could do to add more fat to the foods. She organised vitamins for Mikayla to take each evening to help supplement what she wasn't getting through her diet. Mikayla's tests all came back normal.

Over the next two months we continued with Mikayla's diet and she had some nights with only two to four seizures!! This was truly incredible. She still had the odd busy night with up to ten seizures, but these nights were rare, and still a lot better than the nights of twenty seizures that she had been having.

In July 2017, funding came through for Mikayla to have Stephanie as her dietician for the Modified Atkins Diet. It was a wonderful day.

We started monthly appointments with Stephanie. She would look at Mikayla's food diary and advise where changes needed to be made and how much of each food she could have. Over time we had food charts which showed how much of each food provided one gram of carbohydrate for Mikayla. We found snacks difficult and used the internet to come up with ways of adding fats to snacks and keeping the carbohydrates low. Stephanie advised Mikayla needed to start having Calcium in the morning also in the form of a tablet. Stephanie altered the diet each month, tweaking it here and there until by October she had a daily intake of twenty grams of carbohydrate per day and one hundred and seventy grams of fat.

We saw Dr Hopping from Starship at a clinic appointment in Tauranga in November. She was so happy to see Mikayla looking so well. Not only were her seizures decreasing to no more than eight a night, but she was finally growing and putting on weight. Since April she now weighed forty kilos and had grown ten centimetres. Her cholesterol was quite high, but was dropping from the initial highest level in

June. This was quite common for children on this diet and it usually levelled out over the next year or so. Her hair was even looking more healthy and lush and had stopped falling out. She was getting to school a lot more these days and lasting all day.

"I think it's time to try and reduce some of these medications," she told us. It really was an exciting day. She wrote down how we were to slowly reduce each medication. The weaning off period would take quite some time, but hopefully she would be able to come off some of the medications now that the diet was working fairly well. We started by slowly decreasing the Tegretol, firstly off the morning dose, then the night dose, then back to the morning dose until, eventually, hopefully the Tegretol would be removed. Then we could start on the Clobazam, then Epilim and finally the Acetazolamide.

Meanwhile, Stephanie kept tweaking Mikayla's diet. Adding a little Olivani margarine to her scrambled egg with cream for breakfast one month. Then some almonds to her afternoon tea another month. I had found a recipe for a 'fat bomb' which she ate at lunch and again at afternoon tea, to add some fat to these meals. It consisted of butter, mayonnaise, bacon and hardboiled egg rolled into a truffle ball. At pudding she ate a coconut crème mousse desert, which over the months we got to perfection by adding some coconut oil just before eating.

It was not a cheap diet to be on, but how could you put a price on the type of life we were now having? A child going from twenty or more seizures a night to less than five a night. Mikayla was now having fifty percent seizure free nights! She was growing taller and putting on weight and looking fabulous. She had so much more energy and was enjoying school every day. Dave and I were able to work and we all had so much more energy. No hospital admissions, less respite care, less tests for Mikayla.

Mikayla's twelfth birthday and Christmas were coming up, and we were able to produce a yummy plate of food for her to enjoy with sugar free lollies, chicken nibbles, fat bomb, strawberries with Greek yoghurt, savoury eggs and even a ketogenic birthday cake. Mikayla loved the way she was feeling and the much reduced amount of seizures she was having. She followed the diet perfectly and knew it was so important that she always eat only what we gave her.

In late January 2018, Mikayla started at her new school, Intermediate. She was excited and looked so well walking off to school refreshed and healthy looking. She absolutely loved Intermediate and tried out for many new groups and teams she would never have had the energy to try out for in years gone by. We had weaned her entirely off the Tegretol, and were starting on reducing the Clobazam.

The Intermediate organised a new teacher aide for Mikayla, and she also had the few hours per week with the teacher aide from Northern Health Schools. She was slowly beginning to regain her memory and retention skills at school, and we could begin to teach her things like timetables, which she would never have been able to learn before.

By June, Mikayla had been weaned off the Clobazam and Epilim and was coming off the Acetazolamide. She had a slight increase in seizures on the night we decreased each time, and this would plateau out over the next night or so. Mikayla was seizure free about seventy percent of the nights now and on the other nights would have one to four seizures which were easily managed.

In mid-June we took away Mikayla's last diuretic and she was seizure free for three nights. We thought it was amazing that she had now come off all her medications and the diet was working so well. However, on the fourth night, she had five seizures and on the sixth night she had a terrible night. The seizures occurred every half an hour and they had changed in presentation. She wasn't making the usual panicked sounds we came to recognise with her having a seizure, and it was in fact difficult to hear her. I found her at one point leaning backwards over the dining table, her body convulsing in this position, her face contorted, eyes flickering and she must've been biting her tongue as there was bloodied dribble coming from her mouth. I yelled to Dave, and together we lay her back on the floor, and waited till the seizure stopped. Slowly we got her to her feet. Her poor tongue was all bitten and bleeding, she hadn't done this before. Forty minutes later she had another seizure and bit her tongue again. It was so upsetting to see her doing this to herself I couldn't handle it anymore. I grabbed a blanket and made Mikayla sit up with me watching recorded movies for the rest of the night. If she was awake she couldn't have any seizures so she couldn't damage her tongue any further.

The next night we put the Acetazolamide back in at night and within two nights her seizures had again stopped. It was hard to see her having so many seizures again, and such violent ones at that, but we needed to see what medication she actually needed, and now we knew with the diet, she needed the Acetazolamide at night.

Over the next few months Mikayla's seizures slowly increased again in number with her having up to six or seven some nights. She lost bladder control often too with each seizure. At the end of July she suddenly went very bad slowly increasing over the week to reach twenty five seizures. She was biting her tongue again and losing bladder control with each seizure. We contacted Dr Downing and he suggested adding Acetazolamide in the morning and two hundred milligrams of Epilim at night and perhaps morning also, as it was one of the last medications we had removed. After three nights Mikayla settled down again and by the fourth night of having Acetazolamide and Epilim morning and night her seizures were back down to none most nights with just the odd night of one or two. This combination of diet with a small amount of medication has so far given the best seizure free results for Mikayla.

This brings us to present day, late 2018. Mikayla continues on the Modified Atkins Diet with a small amount of Acetazolamide and Epilim morning and night. She is well controlled now with most night's seizure free and just the odd night with one or two seizures. She is flourishing and looking so healthy and happy. She loves school and is joining in with her class in all events.

We hope that this wonderful result continues for Mikayla. We are hoping that as she gets older they will stop altogether, but the doctors don't know if this will happen or not. We would love the Ketogenic and Modified Atkins Diets to be more readily accessible to children with Epilepsy in New Zealand. At the moment it is up to each District Health Board to get their own funding for dieticians to monitor children on this diet. This is seen as an expensive thing to try, but we feel it is totally worth trying for children with intractable epilepsy. The diet can significantly reduce seizures for up to thirty percent of children, and reduce by at least half the amount of seizures for another thirty percent. Surely this is a huge amount of children and families suffering who could be helped. The cost, we feel, is not justified when you see the suffering a child goes through. The cost of hospital admissions and tests, respite care, teacher aides, in-home care, time off work and school, and personal suffering is just so much larger than trying a child on the diet. It just makes sense.

Aleisha hasn't had a seizure since the one on the cruise ship and we hope that is will be her last one forever.

We are still part of the Genetic Research Trial with the University of Otago. The results came through and Mikayla does carry the gene for nocturnal frontal lobe epilepsy. It was a finding which didn't shock us as all her tests in the hospital had always come back normal. The future of genetics will outline what could be done for Mikayla to perhaps stop her epilepsy for good and prevent it passing onto her children. Aleisha did not have the gene so her seizures were not caused from this. Their biological father, nor I, have the gene either. They told us it's one of those things which can occur during conception.

EPILOGUE

We all take our health for granted. We all take a good night's sleep for granted. Our family will never take either of these things for granted again. To watch someone you love slowly deteriorate and become a shell of who they were. To watch your child who was once so vibrant and cheeky become subdued and weak, with little energy and losing weight. Unable to even go to school or play with her friends. Too tired for outings with family. Childhood memories being forgotten forever due to extreme tiredness and medications. Feeling so tired you feel sick with tiredness. Sleeping with one ear open for your child's next seizure. Suddenly awake, up with your child violently seizing, panicking for breath, making sure they don't hurt themselves. Returning to bed, half asleep, half awake, and waiting for the next seizure to come. Watching the clock tick through the minutes, the hours…yearning for morning to arrive. Then we can get up and stop the seizures…..until the next night comes and you start it all again.

Each medication that is added stops the seizures, if you're lucky for a few days, a few weeks, then the epilepsy fights back, and wins, and you're back again where you were, but with a different list of side effects to deal with. Each morning, you're deciding if she go to school today, can she even get dressed today, can I go to work, can Dave go to work, and do we have the energy to get through the day to day chores that we are meant to. What about our other children and their needs and worries, can we help them and give them what they need, what they deserve. What about us. Us singularly. Us as a married couple. The strain, the worry, the tiredness. Always there……

I hope we are out the other side of this hell. I hope that the diet and medications will continue to provide, if not seizure free nights, then mainly seizure free nights, with nights that we can handle. I hope Mikayla continues to flourish, at school, in health, in life. I hope Aleisha continues to be seizure free. I hope the boys forgive us for being so tired for so long, for being so consumed with getting Mikayla better, for doing the best we could at the time.

I could not have been on this journey without Dave, without family. God brought Dave and I together for love and for strength, through good times and certainly through bad. He is my rock. We have been through hell and he was there for me, for Mikayla, for our children. He sacrificed so much, more than he should've had to. More than most do for marriage…. for love.

I'm not a doctor. I'm not qualified to advise what to do for your child with epilepsy. What worked for Mikayla may not work for your child. What didn't work for Mikayla may work for your child. But follow your gut….. Follow your heart. Talk to your doctor, talk to your paediatrian. They want what's best for your child, for your family.

As Dr Downing always said to us, "controlling Epilepsy is not a science….it is an art," and this is true. You have to try, you have to trust, you have to listen and you have to fight. Read what others have gone through, learn from others mistakes and always have a medical advisor on board with every step you follow. Many people are on the same road as you….many people are on the same journey….we are still on this journey with you…..this is the story of our journey….Mikayla's journey.